# Don't Look Like What I've Been Through

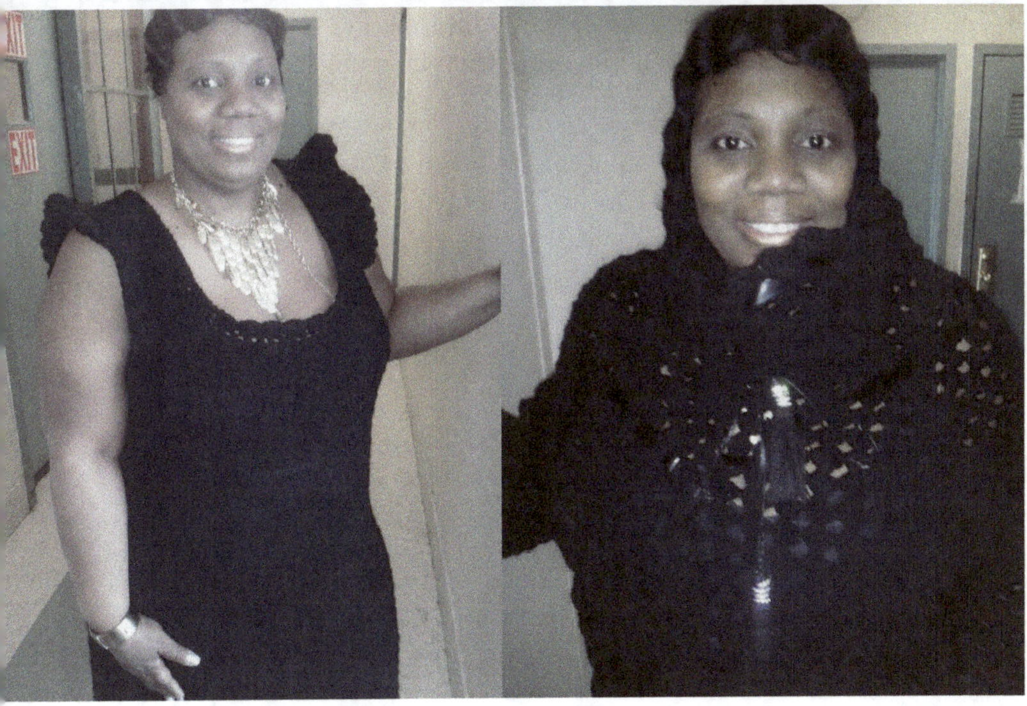

Breaking Free
A Test of Faith and Strength
Memoirs of a Survivor
Copyright © 2015 by Sharon Robinson
ISBN # 978-1-329-43950-4

*Jeremiah 32:27*

*Behold, I am the Lord, the God of all flesh:  Is there anything too hard for me?*

# Special Dedication Page

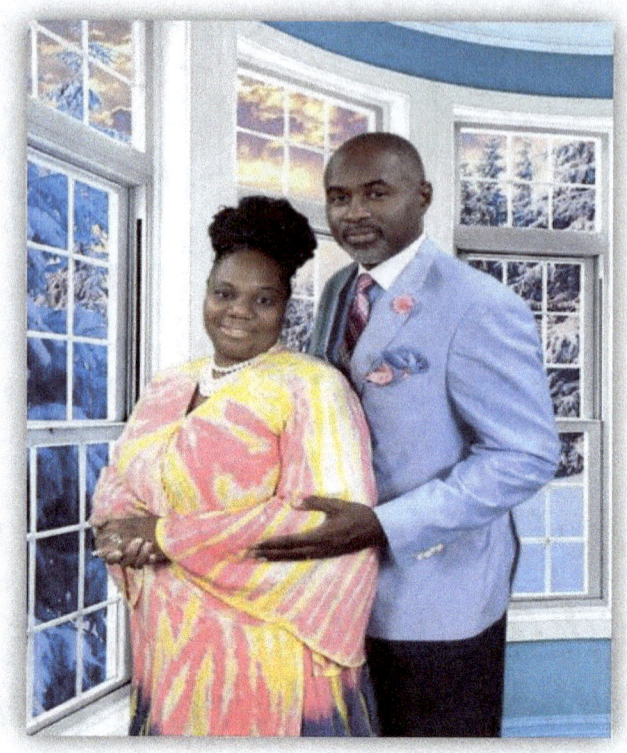

I dedicate this book to my husband of twenty-five (25) years, George and my two (2) sons, George Cameron and Chase Jarrett.

For the past 25 years George has stood the test of time. And there have been some rough times, five miscarriages, one of which were twins, the birth of our two sons, Cameron and Chase one of which I was hospitalized for three months on strict bedrest, laying partially upside down and not being allowed to get out of bed for the entire three months, George was there. We were determined to get our son here by any means necessary. To God be the Glory!! Those times included sick times, colon cancer, breast cancer, chemotherapy treatments, radiation treatments but through it all we did not give up hope we continued to fight to press. I am grateful to God for my husband and for an extraordinary family; I thank God for my sons who were strong and encouraging; my mother, Nelleen Underwood, my mother-in-love Pearl Woods Robinson who were there by my side during my medical ordeal. They were my strength, my inspiration and my prayer warriors!

# Dedication Page

I dedicate this book my best friends Charlene Rivers & family and Elder Michael and Janean Bouie who were all very instrumental in helping me through my medical ordeal.

**Thank You:**
Thank you to my Assistant Pastor, Bishop Charles E. & Mother Faye Wright, Bishop Wilbur L. & Mother Sandra Jones, Elder Reginald & Natalie Brown, my Sister-Girls as I affectionately call them, Dr. Frances L. Hamilton and Ms. Deloris Moore, Ms. Gladys Leonard, my proofreader, my co-workers, Francine Mallozzi, Beatrice Parker and the entire Greater Refuge Temple Family for their prayers and concerns.

I want to especially acknowledge my co-worker, Ms. Francine Mallozzi who I call my office mom; she was such a blessing to me, she attended several of my radiation treatments with me and always had a word of encouragement when I returned to work.

All of you played an active role in keeping me strong.

- Sharon M. Robinson

# The Inspiration

While undergoing my chemotherapy treatment, I felt compelled to write this book to encourage you the reader that no matter what you are going through you can make it. At first I was hesitant but I listened to my heart and obeyed God's voice. I love to write and some time ago I had written a book of poems, had it copyrighted written but never took the necessary steps to get it published.

But this time was different I felt the zeal and the fire to write and publish this book and share my experiences and my testimony. As I began to write this book the words kept flowing and flowing. I had completed chapter one within four days and was amazed at myself and more amazed with God. I knew at that moment that this was supposed to be. When I completed Chapter one, I gave it to my husband to read and when he was done, he had a blank stare on his face. I asked if everything was alright, he responded by saying, "Oh my, this is really good, it's as if I am re-living the moments all over again, you captured every moment". Wow its good he implied.

I want to encourage you the readers to schedule your doctor's appointments, attend them, attend follow-up appointments; listen to the doctors for God gave them the knowledge to help you, eat healthy - eat to live, fight to live and whatever you are going through in your life, most importantly believe God. I want to challenge you to accept this information and allow it to help you from this day forward.

# Acknowledgments

First and foremost I want to give God all the praise and glory for life, strength and enabling me to write this book. I thank God for providing me with wonderful doctors whose compassion, and skills were able to detect a problem and have my situations further evaluated. Through their knowledge and expertise they were able to assist me in my fight against cancer.

I thank God for my mother, Nelleen Underwood and mother-in-love, Pearl Woods-Robinson for their love and support on my journey to recovery. I could not have made it without them. I thank God for the prayers and support from many friends and family.

Words cannot express my sincere appreciation for my medical doctor, Dr. Aryel Nicoleau, my Obstetrician and Gynecologist, Dr. Monique Defour-Jones, the Gastroenterologist, Dr. Ellen Gutkin, the Surgeons, Dr. Litong Du and Dr. James Satterfield of New York Hospital Queens, Member of New York Presbyterian Health Care System, Caroline Rung, Genetic Counselor, Dr. Leonard Farber and the wonderful staff at The Farber Center for Radiation Oncology, my Oncologist Dr. Malvina Fulman and the great Staff at Queens Medical Associates especially my administering nurses, Patricia Holohan and Donna M. Lodato along with Alla Katayev and Nina Ilyayevawho were genuinely concerned and who care so deeply for the patients they serve. Both surgeons as well as the Oncologist were informative and provided me with options which were helpful in my husband's and my decision making.

- Sharon M. Robinson

# TABLE OF CONTENTS

# Faith

Hebrews: 11:1-3

Now **faith** is the substance of things hoped for, the evidence of things not seen. For by it the elders obtained a good report. Through **faith** we understand that the worlds were framed by the word of God, so that things which are seen were not made of things which do appear.

# Chapter 1
## A Test of Faith

*I*t was a cool fall day in October, I remember it so well. My husband, George and I began our normal daily routine as we did every morning. Our days begin early, beginning with getting our sons, George and Chase ready for school. "It's time to get up", I said to the boys as I entered their rooms. "Get up, get up", they began to move slowly as they both rose to get up. As they began to prepare themselves for school, I walked downstairs to the kitchen to prepare breakfast and snacks. After the boys were dressed they hurried into the kitchen to have breakfast. "Your bus will be here soon so let's go", I uttered. Once the boys were done they waited for the school bus, within minutes the bus arrived and off went the boys to school.

It was my husband's and my day off so we climbed back into bed. I prayed that the Lord would bless the day; I had no worries and no concerns. I knew like any other day that all would be well because I serve a mighty God.

After resting a bit, I arose to get ready for my very first colonoscopy. For those of you who are not familiar with a colonoscopy it is as follows:

**What is a Colonoscopy**
[1]A colonoscopy is a test that allows your doctor to examine the inner lining of your large intestine. He or she uses a thin, flexible tube called a colonscope to look at the colon.

A colonoscopy helps to find any: ulcers, colon, polyps, tumors, and areas of inflammation or bleeding. During a colonoscopy tissue samples can be collected (biopsy) and abnormal growth (polyps) can be removed. A Colonoscopy can also be used as a screening test to check for cancer or precancerous growths in the colon or rectum.

**Before the Test**
Before the test you will need to clean out your colon. Colon prep tests take one (1) to two (2) days depending on which type of prep your doctor recommends. Some preps may be taken before the test. The colon prep may be uncomfortable and you may feel hungry because of the liquid diet but hang in there, you can do it!!! I did!! Be sure to drink plenty of water before and after the procedure and follow all instructions.

**Who Gets a Colonoscopy**
[2]Over a million colonoscopies are performed every year in the United States. Most of them are fifty (50) or older to screen for colon cancer. Over eighty (80) percent of the time, the results are normal. When something abnormal is found nine out of ten times it is due to cancer.

Reference: 1webmd; 2about.com

Let me say this before I go on, I am a stickler when it comes to my family's medical and dental appointments. I schedule all the appointments and I even discuss with the doctor certain blood tests that I would like for everyone to have. George and I ask many questions about side effects if any and ask for as much information as possible. I make sure we all have our yearly physicals and follow-up appointments. It is imperative that we as parents, guardians, etc do the same. Early detection is always the best detection. We can learn from what we gain!!

## Hosea 4:6
## My people are destroyed for lack of knowledge…..

Because of my previous physical examination and follow-up appointment, my medical doctor found some abnormalities in my blood work and was concerned that I may be bleeding internally. He wanted me to schedule a colonoscopy for further evaluation. I scheduled the appointment with the Gastroenterologist and really did not give it much thought. I had spoken to several people who had a colonoscopy including my husband and they were fine; their test came back negative. I went with the mind-set that everything was going to be alright.

So off George and I went to my appointment. I was feeling good, blessed and confident; I had no worries or concerns. I knew that God was with me and I believed that the results were going to be negative for me too!!! I took the scripture to heart, as a man thinketh in his heart so is he, so my thoughts were I would have a good report!

## Proverbs 23:7
## For as a man thinketh in his heart so is he………

After the procedure George and I took advantage of our day off. Although I was feeling a bit groggy we managed to do a little shopping, went to lunch and headed home to relax before the boys returned home from school. It was a good day!!! I prayed and stood on God's word as I went about doing my usual routines as a wife, mother, and a help mate to my husband both at home and in the ministry. I often work alongside George in the ministry; I am his secretary and we have worked on several projects together at our church. We are always busy so a little down time for us is always good.

I received a call from my doctor, when the results came back a few days later, informing me that she wanted to meet with me to discuss the results. I felt confident that all was well. George and I met with her and she began by saying (paraphrasing) that my colonoscopy lasted longer than normal. She said she removed several polyps and had sent them to the lab for biopsy and they came back benign. I was relieved. She went on to say that as she was about to complete the procedure she felt compelled to go back and take one last look and in doing so she saw another polyp which seemed to be hidden. She stated that she tried her best to get to it and was unsuccessful as she was about to give up she said she felt a push of her hand and at that moment she was able to grasp a small piece of specimen to send to the lab for biopsy. George and I looked in dismay but we knew it had to be God. I even said to her, that was God. I was not prepared for what she was about to say next at least I thought I was not. She then hit us with the unsuspected news, she said and I quote, "You are a lucky girl". She went on to say that the very last polyp she was able to take a small piece of came back positive for colon cancer. At that moment my heart skipped a beat, "Cancer" I said. She said, "Yes cancer, it appears to be caught in time that is why I said "You are a lucky girl". A slew of emotions had overtaken me, I was stunned and in disbelief. Stunned is what I felt as I heard the diagnosis, I was confused, how could this be? Normally when you hear the word cancer fear overcomes you because of the negative cancer stories you have heard. In some cases fear is what kills many people in this situation - - not the cancer itself;

they give up too soon. And yes I was afraid, but I was stunned more than anything.

I was in disbelief because I never saw this coming. I began this journey feeling good and confident knowing that God was with me and all was going to be well. So again how could this be? My mind was going in all different directions. At one point the doctor was speaking, I saw her lips moving but heard nothing; blah, blah, blah. The doctor saw my facial expression and reassured me that she believed that it was caught in the early stage. After I got over the initial shock, I asked her what stage was it in. I did not want to even say the C-word again. She then informed me that I would have to consult with a surgeon who would inform me at what stage it was in and would schedule more testing to determine what my options would be. She referred me to a surgeon at New York Hospital Queens who was excellent in this field and told me to schedule a consultation as soon as possible. She then stated again that it was caught in time and that early detection is the best detection.

I walked out of her office in dismay. I felt a heavy burden overtake me and I needed to break free; break free from the emotions, break free of the feeling of heaviness, just break free. George and I began to discuss what had just transpired. Still in disbelief I was wondering how I was going to tell this unsuspecting news to my family and close friends. My husband being the calm mannered person he is in crisis suggested that it would be best to meet with the surgeon first, get all of the necessary information and see what my options were going to be before we share the news. I agreed. Although I could not understand why this was happening to me, I needed to put on the garment of praise for the heaviness I was feeling.

## Isaiah 61:3

**To appoint unto them that mourn in Zion, to give unto them beauty for ashes, the oil of joy for mourning, the garment of praise for the spirit of heaviness..**

## Matthew 11:28

**Come unto me, all ye that labour and are heavy laden, and I will give you rest.**

Let me interject here, in life we all will be faced with many stumbling blocks, but God can
    1) Remove the stumbling block,
    2) Help you over the stumbling block and/or
    3) Remove the stumbling block completely. He can even do all three at the same time,
        that is the kind of God He is.

## Isaiah 57:14

**And shall say, Cast ye up, cast ye up, prepare the way, take up the stumbling block out of the way of my people.**

You see sometimes we are set-up for the stumbling blocks; but your set-ups are designed for come-backs. Here I was in a set-up, facing a stumbling block. How was I going to come out of this? Was I going to come out of this? I didn't even know where to begin, I could not pray! I needed to put on the garment of praise for this heaviness and at the moment I could not do it. I felt alone, I felt betrayed. I remembered a sermon my former pastor, Bishop Wilbur L, Jones preached some time ago, "Stored Up Prayers" which basically explained how there may come a time in your life when you cannot pray and you need to pray continually and store up your prayers for difficult times. Those of you who are reading this, have you ever been there? Well my God, I was there I was at that point! I tried to pray and the devil brought to my mind how I believed God and how I thought God was with me. He said, Where is God Now"? My mind was racing and I thought to myself, God have you forgotten about me? Did you leave me? I got no reply. This went on for a few days, I began to keep quiet and still. One night my husband came into the room where I was sitting, he said to me "Babe whatever the outcome, He didn't believe that God would bring us this far and leave us". He believed that all was going to be alright.

With that in mind, I called and scheduled a consultation with the surgeon at the New York Hospital Queens. Within a few days my husband and I met with the surgeon. We both prayed that whatever the outcome we would together believe God for healing and deliverance. The surgeon began discussing the pathology report and reviewing the pathology film with us. He reiterated that I indeed had colon cancer. I sat there baffled all over again! He wanted to know what made my doctor schedule me for a colonoscopy at my age since I was not yet fifty. I explained to him that it was determined after I had my physical examination. My medical doctor saw some abnormalities in my blood work and decided that I needed to schedule a colonoscopy for further testing to ensure that I was not bleeding internally. The doctor replied that I had a very good medical doctor who was very thorough. He then said something that struck me and George. He said he was amazed that the Gastroenterologist found the small tumor.  He stated that where the tumor was located it was hidden and he was surprised that she was able to find it.  He implied by the time the tumor would have been detected it would have been too late for me.  "Look at God"!  My heart began to race, I murmured in a calm voice, it was God and he responded yes it was.  At that moment I knew God was with me; He did not leave me.  God had spoken back to me through the doctor.

## Deuteronomy 31:6
### Be strong and courageous. Do not be afraid or terrified because of them, for the LORD your God goes with you; he will never leave you nor forsake you."

You see God has a way of showing up when you least expect Him to.  He has a way of letting you know He is with you.  God will place the right people in your path that will help you; the team of doctors were placed in my life to help me.  I was told that I had to undergo surgery to remove the cancerous tumor in order for the cancer not to return, it was his recommendation to remove the entire right colon.  The surgeon stated in doing this there is a 99.8% chance that the cancer will not return.  He stated that he would have to reconstruct my colon so that I would be able to move my bowels on my own without a colostomy bag.  He went on to say that before the actual surgery date I would have to undergo a series of tests, preferably a Cat-Scan (C-Scan) and a Magnetic Resonance Imaging (MRI).  These tests are performed to look more closely at the cancerous tumor which will determine how they were going to deal with the tumor once they perform the surgery.  He said that once he is performing the surgery he will then be able to determine what stage the cancer was and if the cancer had spread.

Through the entire extremely uncomfortable test and the waiting for the actual surgery, I was very anxious; I wanted it to all be over. Once the test results came back and we had a better understanding of what my options were, I was cleared to have surgery and wanted to have it as soon as possible. If I could have had it that day I would have. It was around the Christmas holiday and I wanted to have the surgery before the New Year. I remember asking the doctor if the surgery can take place before the New Year and he said, "No after the New Year". He told me to enjoy the holidays!! How could I, I thought to myself. It seemed as though a long time had passed and in all of my anxiousness I wanted it over. I know the bible speaks of being anxious,

## Philippians 4:6
## Be anxious for nothing: but in everything by prayer and supplication with thanksgiving let your requests be made known unto God

But I could not help it, I was anxious after all it's easier said than done. Even in my anxious state, I had to honestly learn to trust God; I can truly say it was not easy. In all my forty years of being a Christian, I thought I had it all together; I thought my faith was up to par. But when you are in a state of sickness or your back is against a wall is when you learn where your faith really lies. You have to learn how to really trust God and totally lean and depend on Him for healing. Once you decide to take that leap of faith and totally lean on God for healing you must first believe that God can heal. How can you have faith if you don't believe? I had to lean on God in my situation even if I had to work through chemotherapy, radiation or whatever the doctors recommended. I had to put my entire being in

God's hand and trust Him. Again I say it was easier said than done though; I had to constantly speak life to myself and stir up the Word that was in me. I had to allow God to guide my mind and the hands of the doctors who were working on my behalf.

Sometimes as Christians we think we have so much faith in Him. Until you are in an actual situation is when you learn how much faith you really have. Now I am not saying that it's all Christians, some Christians have more faith than others and some of us have to go through a process so that our faith in Him can be increased. That was me! Some of us are placed in situations so that we can learn who God really is and what He can do if we "Trust Him". God will be with you through whatever you are facing.

## Proverbs 3:5-6
### 5Trust in the Lord with all thine heart; and lean not unto thine own understanding.
### 6In all thy ways acknowledge him, and he shall direct thy paths.

Once I received the surgery date and had a better understanding of my diagnosis and what was going to take place during surgery, we were better equipped to share the news with our family and close friends. I was very reluctant to tell my mother, after all she is my mother and I am her daughter and her only child. I knew it was going to be hard for me to say and her to accept. When I finally shared the news with her she paused a moment, I can tell she was trying to be strong for me. She then replied, "Whose report do you believe, believe the report of the Lord". She mentioned that was the sermon her pastor, Bishop Wilbur L. Jones preached the previous Sunday. Look how God works; He will prepare you for what is to come. I detected that my mom was worried but both she and I stood on the Word, "Whose report do you believe, believe the report of the Lord". George and I then had to share the news with my mother in-love, when we told her she too paused. Her statement to us was, "If you are going to worry why pray and if you are going to pray why worry". She said that God was in control and that she felt everything was going to be alright.

Why are you sharing all of this Sharon? If you are reading this I proclaim that whatever you are going through you needed to read this! Perhaps you too may have received a bad report from the doctor or bad news from your lawyer; it is high time to pray and not worry and to believe the report of the Lord. You are coming out of your current situation with more faith than you ever had. But in order to do so you must not only say it, you must believe it. Don't just say it, you must act on it.

I became more open to God and more trusting in Him. That night and many nights thereafter I went into my secret closet, I know many of you know what I am talking about; I laid prostrate on my face before God in prayer. At first I could not utter any words out of my mouth; all I could do was cry and moan. Thank God he understands every moan and groan. I laid there until my breakthrough came; I placed my hand on my abdomen and continued to cry and moan. I lay before God until I could feel strength come into my body and a burning in my belly. I was able at that point to open my mouth and pray these words to God, "Lord I put my body in your hands, Lord I feel your touch". Hallelujah! I heard God's voice so clear, "I am with you, I will never leave you". From that point on, I took comfort in knowing that God was with me, He was my strength; the strength that is different from the strength of a spouse or a family member. It is the strength that gives you comfort that everything was going to be alright; the strength to go on. God is an awesome God!! I would like to encourage you to trust Him in every aspect of your life.

## The Surgery

My surgery day had finally arrived. The night before the surgery I received a call from my Assistant Pastor and his wife, Bishop Charles E. Wright and Mother Faye Wright who wanted to have prayer with me and the family before the surgery, God moved in a mighty way. I felt uplifted and felt that all was going to be well. God had even given me sweet sleep that night; I had slept through the night.

### Jeremiah 31:26
### ….. and my sleep was sweet unto me.

However, when I awoke in the morning about a half hour before I was going to get up to prepare to go to the hospital for the surgery, I can remember it was a cold January day in 2013 and I was overcome by fear, nervousness and had such an uneasy feeling because it was the big day. During that half hour I tossed and turned and I began to pray and ask God to take away the uneasy feeling. As I uttered this request, the telephone rang, it was my good friends, my brother and sister, Elder and Sister Michael and Janean Bouie. They called to have prayer with me and the family and to intercede on my behalf before the surgery that morning. The prayers of the righteous availeth much.

### James 5:16
### Confess your faults one to another, and pray
### one for another, that ye may be healed. The

## effectual fervent prayer of a righteous man availeth much.

Elder Bouie prayed these words into my spirit, "God take away any uneasy spirit that Sharon may be experiencing right now, help her to be still and know that you are God, you are the healer, you are the way maker, Lord touch her infirmities, touch the hands of the surgeon and remove all doubt and feelings of discouragement in the name of Jesus".   My God, my God how did Elder Bouie know what I was feeling, what a mighty God we serve.  God's timing is always right.  By the time he was done, the feeling lifted and George and I were praising God.   What is so ironic about this situation is that Elder Bouie tried calling me the night before and I was not available to speak with him at the time. God knew what I was going to go through the next morning and sent him as an intercessor. After George and I were ready to leave for the hospital, I informed my mother that we were getting ready to leave and she remarked that I was quite bubbly and chipper.  My words to her were, "I am going to be alright mom, all is well".  She said amen!!  I had reached that point where I had to believe God and take responsibility for doing whatever is physically possible to ensure my health.

For believers and non-believers there are going to be times in your life when situations may arise and you have to be still and quiet. It is those times you should seek guidance from God and ask that the eyes of your understanding be enlightened so that you may make the right decisions.  It is also that moment you should ask yourselves honestly, is this the life I want to live without the presence of God?  I invite you to allow God to be God in those yet still moments.

## Psalm 46:10
**Be still, and know that I am God: I will be exalted among the heathen, I will be exalted in the earth.**

Allow me to briefly discuss the words be still; Be still can mean not moving and being quiet. So many times as believers we ask God for things but we don't stop to listen or be still long enough for Him to speak to us or He speaks and we are so busy moving about that we do not hear Him. We are shaped by this hectic world we live in where everything is so fast paced. We need to slow down and rewind. God wants us to **BE STILL** so that we can receive the peace and guidance we need to make it through and make the right decisions. When you take the time to be still you will see your attitude change, you will become calmer and God can then work the way He wants to work in your life and in your situation. God will guide your steps and give you peace.

## Numbers 6:26
**The Lord lift up his countenance upon thee, and give thee peace.**

I can go on and on because God is so good. I thank God for surrounding me with praying people who can pray peace into my life; peace into my situation. I thank God for a praying husband, praying parents, my Assistant Pastor, Bishop Charles E. Wright, praying friends, Elder and Sister Michael Bouie and Charlene Rivers and a praying church family, I am truly blessed. The prayers of the righteous truly availeth much. I went into surgery knowing that I was going to be alright, I was going to be cancer free. God had spoken, "Be still, I am God". God was with me.

As I waited to be called to be prepped for surgery, I was calm and I was still; let me explain my spirit was still. I had to continue to encourage myself while I waited. George said to me, "Babe, it's going to work out you'll see" as he uttered a prayer. I was then called to be prepped for the surgery. Once I lay on the table to undergo surgery I can remember the anesthesiologist conversing with me. Before I went completely out I can remember saying thank you Jesus.

"Mrs. Robinson, Mrs. Robinson, you are in the recovery room wake up" spoke the recovery nurse. I slowly opened my eyes and there stood my husband by my side holding my hand. I tried to move and oh the pain, my entire body seemed to hurt. I was so uncomfortable. George stood there gazing at me and asked how I was feeling. I said, "In PAIN!!! Moments later the surgeon came into my section of the recovery room and pulled the curtains, he began to discuss the results of the surgery. He smiled and stated that the surgery went very well and that it seemed as though the cancer was caught in time and had not spread. He implied that he was able to reconstruct my colon and that I did not need a colostomy bag. He said that he would be able to confirm all of his findings once the pathology report is back in a few days. As I lay there I began to thank God for what he had done and for the Victory report. I was in the hospital for three (3) days and during those days I would spend my day praying and thanking God for complete healing. One day while sitting in the chair preparing myself to go for my walk down the halls of the hospital for exercise, I began to sing this song: **Victory ahead, victory ahead, through the blood of Jesus,**

**victory ahead, trusting in the Lord, I hear the conqueror say, by faith I see the victory ahead!**

Although I was in great pain, I was encouraged. I did not allow the hospital bed to consume me; I began walking the halls of the hospital several times a day each day humming the song of victory. The nurses were amazed; they commented that they wished their patients were more like me because most patients who are in pain do not want to move let alone walk around. I refused to just lie there and become stiff so I walked every chance I received; I must admit the morphine medication helped move me along too!!! ☺ I prayed and sang and had a good time just me and Jesus. I got up early in the morning to wash and prepare for breakfast which was very early and after breakfast I would slowly walk the halls. As I walked the halls I began to pray not only for myself but for the other patients around me. I received visits from some of my good friends who prayed with me. Through my prayers and the prayers of others I gained my strength each day. One day as I was talking to the patient in the next bed, she said to me you must be a popular girl, you always have visitors and they are always praying for you. Do you think they will pray for me? Wow I thought to myself, as I mentioned to her that yes indeed they will pray for you and with you. When my husband who is a deacon of our church at The Greater Refuge Temple came that evening, we had pray with her and asked God to touch her body and bless her family. When he left for the evening she said that she never had anyone pray for her like that before and she felt good. I was so thankful to God that we were able to pray with and for her. I asked her if I could have her telephone number so that we could keep in contact with each other and she said certainly so we exchanged numbers. I felt good. I was meant to be in the hospital room with her. Glory Be to God!!

I was truly encouraged. Once the pathology report was back, the surgeon met with George and I and the victory report was confirmed. I was cancer free with a 99.8% chance that it will not return. Glory Be to God! Things were looking up. He then referred me to an oncologist and asked me to schedule a consultation with her to discuss the possibility of chemotherapy and/or radiation. God had begun the process of healing and He had to finish what He had started. He who begun a good work.....

### Philippians 1:6
**Being confident of this very thing, that he which hath begun a good work in you will perform it until the day of Jesus Christ:**

God had begun the healing process and He had to complete it, that's His Word. Glory Be to God!! I did not want my faith to be shaken; I decreed that I was not going to have chemo-therapy and/or radiation. I believed that God was going to complete His work in me.

George and I met with the oncologist who was very pleasant and caring. She reviewed the report and basically repeated what the surgeon had previously stated. She then said what I was waiting to hear, Chemotherapy and/or radiation was NOT recommended but that it was her recommendation that I have a colonoscopy every six (6) months for observation. I was rejoicing and singing *Victory is Mine* and giving God all the praise.

After going through the colon cancer surgery, recuperating and seeing my oncologist, I continued praising God for the victory. I visited my Gastroenterologist for my six month check-up and I was ecstatic when she informed me that I was cancer free. Thank You Jesus!!! God is so good! Hallelujah!

When you are going through sickness or life's trials, it can be difficult to believe God. I am a witness!! Your faith is put on trial and your faith can be shaken, but you must hold fast the profession of your faith without wavering.

## Hebrews 10:23
### Let us hold fast the profession of our faith without wavering; for he is faithful that promise.

If God said it, that settles it! Let me ask, how many of you have flown before? You put your faith and trust in the pilot who you don't know to get you to your destination safely. You run into turbulence and still you sit in your seat some praying others nervous but you don't give up and walk off a moving plane; you have faith that you will arrive to your destination safely. If you can put your faith in a pilot whom you don't know, how can you not put your trust in the one who gave you life? God even prepares the way for you when the turbulences of life come your way. God will set you up to be blessed. Hallelujah!!!

Allow me to take a moment to explain faith, you see faith is a firm conviction in the accomplishment of something; the confidence that one's expectation will be met and fulfilled. We must feed ourselves with words of faith. A man or woman holding on to something never falls, the only time they may fall is if they let go. You need to hold fast to something. I encourage you to grab a hold to God and don't let Him go.  Don't you dare let go; don't you dare give up.  **HOLD ON!!**

No matter what you are going through or what the enemy places in front of you, it is important for you to hold fast the profession of your faith.  Do not give up half way through your mission; you will be alright if you hold fast. The closer one gets to complete the mission the more you feel you want to give up.  But I encourage you to believe in the possibilities not the problem; your mission is almost complete.

Perhaps you are reading this and thinking it is easier said than done, I am a witness.  Some of you have reached that point in your life where you want to give up but you can't, not now, you are too close to victory.  Stretch forth your FAITH and put it into action.  Hold fast, cling to your faith even when everything looks dreary.   Don't you dare let go!!!  "I sure did not".  I can personally assure you that God's Word works and He can meet you right where you are and help you in your time of need.

It was not easy for me to hold on, at times I said why me. But through this test my faith became strong.  I have seen what God can do.   If he can do it for me, He can surely do it for you my friend.

# Strength

Isaiah 40:29
He giveth power to the faint; and to them that have no
might he increaseth **strength**.

# Chapter 2
## A Test of Strength

After my colon cancer ordeal, I was feeling blessed, my faith was increased, I was feeling good and even more confident. I knew that God was with me and I felt so elated that God had bought me through the test without having to have chemotherapy or radiation. It was my test and I had passed the test, my faith in God was increased and I knew there was nothing I could not do because God was on my side. I praised God and continued to praise God for the experience, and I was moving forward with my life. I looked at life a little differently, I served God in a way I never served before, I trusted Him, I believed Him, I loved God more. I loved my husband, sons and family even more. They were who I wanted to live for. I loved my family; they were my prayer warriors; the ones who called the most to give me encouragement and to offer a word prayer and loved my friends more because they stood by my side and were there for me and my family.

I thank God for allowing me to go through this test. What I have learned had been a sure test of faith. The battle I was going through was not mine, but God's. I had to let God fight this battle, the battle in my body and the battle of my mind.

**II Chronicles 20:15**
**....for the battle is not yours, but God's.**

God tells Jehoshaphat in II Chronicles 20:15 that the battle was not his but it was God's. Just like he told Jehoshaphat this, God reminded me that I was not alone in this battle; in other words, "He's got this". Although it was a physical problem, God was going to work it out in the spiritual realm. The Holy Spirit and God's spirit had to connect and I had to focus on God and not the physical problem. I had to let God handle it and stand firm on Him. God is much better at fighting our battles much better than you or I could ever be; God has never lost a battle. Our job is to trust God at His Word and believe that He can do what He said He could do. God told Jehoshaphat and tells us today to take our rightful position and that is -- to **STAND** firm on Him. So having done all, you just **STAND**.

## Ephesians 6:13
**Wherefore take unto you the whole armour of God, that ye may be able to withstand in the evil day, and having done all, to STAND.**

**Strength In This Present Hour**
It was the summer of 2013 I lay in bed preparing to go to sleep for the night. I began to do a self-breast examination as I did periodically. As I am examining my breast, I felt a small lump in my right breast. I did get a little excited but remembered that I have what is called Fibrocystic breast. Because of the cystic breast, I began having mammogram testing at an early age.

**¡What Are Fibrocystic Breasts**
This topic covers breast changes that feel lumpy, thick, and tender before your menstrual period. It is not meant for women who have had a breast biopsy showing "atypia" or

"hyperplasia." These are cell changes that may lead to cancer.

**What are fibrocystic breast changes?**
Many women have breasts that feel lumpy, thick, and tender, especially right before their periods. These symptoms are called fibrocystic breast changes. They may also be called cyclic breast changes because they come and go with your menstrual cycle.
Fibrocystic breast changes are normal and harmless. They are not cancer, and they do not increase your chance of getting breast cancer.

But having fibrocystic breast changes can make it harder to find a lump that could be cancer. This is a special concern if you also have a higher than normal risk for breast cancer. So if you or a close family member has had breast cancer or if you have had radiation treatment or a breast biopsy showing atypical ductal hyperplasia (ADH), talk to your doctor about how often you need a breast checkup.

**What is a Mammography**
1A mammography is an x-ray examination of the breast used to detect and diagnose breast disease. Mammography is the most effective method of detecting cancer at an early stage. Screening mammography is used as a preventive measure for women who have no symptoms of breast disease. A screening mammography usually involves views of each breast.

The very next morning I called my doctor immediately and informed her of what I had felt and a mammography was scheduled the same week. I have a yearly mammography and like any other year I did not worry too much because I knew I had cystic breast and in the past all my mammograms were negative. Two days after my mammography, I received a call from the technician who informed me that there were some inconsistencies in my exam and that I needed to retake the examination. So off I went once again to take another exam. Again I was not concerned, I felt like everything was ok. A day later I received a call from my OB/GYN doctor, Dr. Monique Defour-Jones informing me that she wanted me to schedule a sonogram so that she can get a clearer view of my right breast. At that point, I became a little suspicious because this had never happened before. What is going on I thought to myself, Lord is my strength in you on trial, I uttered to myself.

I needed some renewed strength for this was becoming a little too much.

### Isaiah 40:31
**But they that wait upon the Lord shall renew their strength; they shall mount up with wings as eagles; they shall run, and not be weary; and they shall walk and not faint.**

After the sonogram, I met with my doctor to discuss the results and to my surprise, she muttered those words I did not want to hear, "You have breast cancer". I was startled, I did not understand why, I did not know if I wanted to sob or scream but refused to do either. My head began to hurt as I sat there in total disbelief. Here we go again I thought to myself. Having gone through my first battle with colon cancer, I thought I was done. You see I've learned that things happen in seasons I thought my season of sickness had come and gone. But I was dreadfully wrong.

Reference: 1JohnHopkinsMedicine.com; WEBMD

### Ecclesiastes 3:1-3

**1To everything there is a season, and a time to every purpose under the heaven: 2A time to be born, and a time to die; a time to plant, and a time to pluck up that which is planted; ….3and a time to heal; a time to break down, and a time to build up; ......**

Here it is five months later the "C" word is mentioned again. As I left her office, I did not know where or how to begin to tell my husband. I had told him to go to work that day because I was not expecting to hear this kind of news. As I was walking to my car the words of Tye Tibbett's song began to ring in my head, "If He Did It Before, He Can Do It Again". When I started my car and turned on the radio, guess what was playing, yes that song. That song stayed with me through the entire ordeal.

That evening after my sons went to bed for the night I discussed with George what the doctor had informed me. He looked puzzled and shocked. He said in a calm voice, "Sharon, everything is going to be alright, "If He Did It Before, He Will Do It Again? Glory Be to God that was confirmation.

As I sat there I said to my husband you know, **Weeping is not an option** for me,

### Psalm 30:5

**....weeping may endure for a night, but joy cometh in the morning.**

**Depression is not an option** for me,

**Isaiah 26:3**
**Thou wilt keep him in perfect peace, whose mind is stayed on thee: because he trusteth in thee.**

**Sickness is not an option** for me,
**I Peter 2:24**
**Who his own self bare our sins in his own body on the tree, that we, being dead to sins, should live unto righteousness: by whose stripes ye were healed.**

I thank and praise God for His Word; His Word can comfort you in your darkest hour. I also thank God for my husband, he is always so calm in the face of adversity and that helps to keep me calm too. He is such a blessing to our family. Some husbands would have said enough is enough and walked away, but he has stood by my side literally through sickness and health. Our wedding vows had really come alive and he took them very seriously, to be there for me in sickness and health. Thank you Jesus!

I was referred to a surgeon who was excellent in this field. George and I met with the surgeon, Dr. James Satterfield who discussed and reviewed the sonogram report and pictures with us. He confirmed the diagnosis of breast cancer and scheduled a Biospy, MRI and CatScan to further confirm the findings as well as determine which option would be best for my situation.  Dr. Satterfield was very caring and supportive to both my George and I.

All of the news was an unexpected shock to me.  I was hoping it was not cancer but a cyst or something, anything but cancer.  I had to wait on the results of the test to determine what kind of surgery I would need; will it be a lumpectomy and mastectomy?  I had to wait until after the surgery to determine what stage the cancer was in and see if the cancer had spread.

When you are going through the test of life you have to encourage yourself as I have done in time past.  Once again I had to speak God's Word into my spirit. I told myself, "This Sickness is Not Unto Death, for I Will Live and Not Die".

## John 11:4

**When Jesus heard that, he said, This sickness is not unto death, but for the glory of God, that the Son of God might be glorified thereby.**

Through all of the series of tests, I was not as anxious this time, this time was a little different.  I was somewhat at peace and believed God for my healing whichever way it came.   God can perform a miracle or God can use the doctor.  I declared once again that I would live and **NOT** die. I was in God's hand and my trust was in Him.  George and I trusted God and we staggered not, we stood in faith together that God was going to see me through once again. Once again George was my strength, God supplied the strength we needed and He was our source.  What God has promised He will do; I had to once again trust in God.

## Romans 4:20
**He staggered not at the promise of God through unbelief; but was strong in faith, giving glory to God.**

God will give you the strength, the faith, the fight, the zeal to live but you have to have a mind to do so. You never know the STRENGTH you have until you are in a test. You see, in my previous test, my faith in God was increased. I had a better understanding of having faith and putting faith into action. Faith had become an action not inaction to me.

## Mark 11:22
**And Jesus answering saith unto them, Have faith in God.**

Not only did I have to learn to put my faith in God, I had to believe that what I asked God for that He would bring it to pass. I literally had to trust and take God at His word. In order to receive the blessings from God, you have to do something. Faith, believing and trusting all go hand in hand.

## Mark 11:23
**For verily I say unto you, That whosoever shall say unto this mountain, Be thou removed, and be thou cast into the sea; and shall not doubt in his heart, but shall believe that those things which he saith shall come to pass; he shall have whatsoever he saith.**

We cannot take our eyes off of God; we must continue to move forward. God will keep His promise as long as you keep your PRAISE. Praise brings forth Victory, Faith brings forth Strength and Strength brings forth Hope. I remained hopeful because of my strength and faith in God.

Now here comes the hard part, I had to once again tell this unexpected news to my family and close friends. Oh how do I tell this!! I began by telling my mother, she was in shock she blurted "Oh no Sharon". She proclaimed yet again, "Whose report do you believe, believe the report of the Lord". I echoed, "Oh yes I believe the report of the Lord". I will live and I will not die for this is not unto death. She uttered the words, "This too shall pass". I said amen, I receive that. We then told my mother-in-love and she too said yet again "If you are going to worry why pray and if you are going to pray why worry". I said to her you are absolutely right because if God did it before, He can do it again and again and again. I told her I was going to be alright. She said to me, "Sharon you are so encouraging, so strong, my hat's off to you, and yes you are going to be alright". What would I do without my parents? They have been my prayer warriors, I thank God for them.

The summer days seemed longer and hotter than usual. George and I were in a dilemma, we were not sure if we wanted to go on vacation because of my situation. I was still under the doctor's care and currently awaiting test results. While sitting at work one day, my best friend and sister, Charlene called and said these words to me, "Sharon you need a vacation after all the hell you have gone through this year, you need to get away to clear your head". She went on to say that one of the airlines was offering discounted tickets and that we must purchase them right away. I called my husband immediately to discuss it. After which I called my doctor, Dr. Satterfield to verify if I could travel and he said, yes by all means I should go on vacation and enjoy myself with my family.

My test results were not back before we went on vacation and we had planned to leave for Orlando, Florida that Sunday afternoon. My doctor told me to contact his office on Tuesday to ascertain the results. I was excited to be going on a well-deserved vacation with my family and close friends. While on vacation my plan was to try not to dwell too much on my situation and as Charlene mentioned take the time to away to pray and clear my head. I thank God for my sister and friend. She indeed is a blessing to me and my family.

We were having a great time and I was really enjoying myself. That Tuesday while still away on vacation as requested by the doctor I called to see if the results were back and to my surprise the doctor had been called into emergency surgery and therefore I had to wait another day for the results. I really believe that God put me in the position to wait to teach me some things. I began to see things differently and a little more clearly. I was being taught to wait and while waiting PRAY!! Waiting can be very difficult because you want it NOW, I don't like to wait, but I had no choice I had to wait. I thought about a scenario involving waiting. Picture it, you are waiting on a bus in the cold icy weather, you stand there feeling cold, your nose getting numb, chattering your teeth, but you are looking for the bus in anticipation that it would come sooner than later. You wait squirming and fidgeting restlessly trying to keep warm; hoping and wishing the bus would come. Like waiting for the bus, I wanted my answer from the doctor sooner; I wanted it on Tuesday when I called. Sometimes we wait on God the same way, we squirm, and we fidget restlessly and want God to answer us sooner than later. We want the answer NOW, the healing

NOW, the blessing NOW. But God makes us wait because He is molding us and teaching us who He really is and what He can do while we wait. God is not the bus driver, He's not us standing in the cold waiting for the bus to come He is God; He is waiting on us. God can show you some amazing things while you're waiting and abiding in Him for your healing, for your blessing.

## Psalm 40:1
## I waited patiently for the Lord; and he inclined unto me, and heard my cry.

I advise you the reader to learn to wait on God and while you wait PRAY. God is an awesome God; He is listening and waiting on you.

I called the doctor the next day and yet again he was not available. No matter how it looks, you have to see the good in situations and try not to dwell on negativity. Although I could not reach my doctor I began to take this as a good sign that all was going to be well. While I waited I went into prayer mode even on vacation and laid prostrate on my face before God yet again for my healing. Lord I thank you for the wait.

That Friday morning I was awakened out of my sleep at 9am and was compelled to call the doctor right then. I knew I was taking a chance calling his office because on Fridays he is normally in surgery most of the day and rarely in the office. Because I was compelled to call I did so and to my surprise he was in the office. I really should not have been surprised because it was all in God's plan. I can remember the office administrator telling me that I had just caught the doctor because he was about to leave to return to the hospital. God is good! I spoke to the doctor and he informed me that the test results were back and that the Biospy concluded that it was breast cancer. I then asked him what would he recommend in my situation and he replied that this was his field of expertise and would recommend that I have a Lumpectomy. He said he had done many of these procedures in the past and because of his expertise and my positive attitude I was going to be fine. I thank God for those words of encouragement from my doctor. When George had awakened later on that morning I shared the news with him and he reassured me that all was going to be well.

Lumpectomy

Copyright © 2001 WebMD Corporation

### 2What is a Lumpectomy

Lumpectomy is also called breast-conserving surgery. The surgeon removes the tumor and a little bit of healthy tissue around it. A second incision under the armpit may be made to remove the lymph nodes. The goal of a lumpectomy is to leave as much of your healthy breast tissue alone as possible. After the lumpectomy, radiation is usually used to treat any cancer cells that were left behind.

Lumpectomies are best for women who have small, early-stage breast cancers.
Some women shouldn't get a lumpectomy:
- Women who have already had radiation for their breast cancer
- Women who have two or more areas of cancer in the same breast that are too far apart to be removed through one incision
- Women who have large tumors

If you have a large tumor, sometimes you can get chemotherapy or hormone therapy to shrink it first, and then have a lumpectomy.

Despite the news I continued to enjoy the rest of my vacation. I refused to be depressed or upset because I knew that God was going to see me through this. I had to continue to move forward regardless of what it seemed like. God had known my situation and the outcome even before I had spoken to the doctor. I knew I was going to be made whole. What is the meaning of "Whole"? Well the Webster's II New College Dictionary defines "Whole" as sound, healthy, restored. It would imply complete restoration of body parts that were diseased or unhealthy. God can remove the unhealthy thing and restore your health. He can use the doctors to do so or He is well capable of performing a miracle. You can and will be made "WHOLE", take that devil!!

## Luke 8:50
### But when Jesus heard it, he answered him saying, Fear not: believe only, and she shall be made whole.

My God is an awesome God; His words are so genuine, so clear, so real. "WHOLE", Speak Lord! God's Word truly sustained me. I will be made "WHOLE" and restored to good health.

Upon my return from vacation, I came home with a clear head. I was more uplifted and ready to face my test and allow God to have his way in me and through me. I drew my strength from God's word and my husband who remained positive and hopeful. I wanted God to be glorified in my situation which I had learned in my first fight with colon cancer.

In the midst of it all I remember getting a call from one of my friends who knew my situation and what she was getting ready to say I needed to hear. She asked a question; one in which I never wondered really about, did I know the difference between Affliction and Sickness, I said yes, she then elaborated on the difference between the two.

Reference: 2WebMD.com
Merriam-Webster.com

**What is Sickness** (Paraphrasing)

Sickness is the condition of being sick; illness. You know in your body that the sickness exists and spiritually you have to focus on the inner state of being, the sickness is there but God is able to heal.


## Exodus 15:26
## ... For I am the Lord that healeth thee.


## Exodus 23:25
## And ye shall serve the Lord your God, and he shall bless thy bread, and thy water; I will take away sickness away from the midst of thee.


"It is not nearly as important what disease the patient has as to what patient has the disease." -- Sir William Osler put it so eloquently. Are you the patient who dwells on the disease and soak in your sorrows or are you that patient who hears that they have the disease push pass what you have heard and believe that you are going to get through with God's help. Which category do you fall into? I was that patient who heard the news and even in my state of mind did not allow myself to submit to the disease but to submit the disease to God for my healing.

**What is Affliction**

Affliction is the terrorization of the mind, body and soul. It makes your mind wonder about the "What-Ifs"; oh no I have cancer **what if** I suffer, **what if** I die, you wonder about your family—what would happen to them if you are not around and the most famous one, Why Me? At one point I had reached that place where I asked God why me too! But once I overcame the fact that I was in my struggle I began to believe that I was going to be made "WHOLE". I then boasted in God and replied "Why Not Me, Here Am I God Use Me in This Struggle". I realized that this struggle had to exist so that I could be an example for you and to let you know that you are not alone, God is with you. If you are in a struggle think positively and do not allow the enemy to eat away at your mind. Begin to think that you will be made "Whole" in whatever situation you are facing. Change your thought pattern and think on the things that are lovely. Keep your mind on God not the situation.

**Philippians 4:8**
**Finally, brethren, whatsoever things are true, whatsoever things are honest, whatsoever things are just, whatsoever things are pure, whatsoever things are lovely, whatsoever things are of a good report; if there be any virtue, and if there be any praise, think on these things.**

**II Corinthians 10:5**
**Casting down imaginations, and every high thing that exalteth itself against the knowledge**

**of God, and bringing into captivity every thought to the obedience of Christ.**

Although we walk in the flesh we do not war after the flesh. We must cast down every negative imagination. I know it's easier said than done but I am a witness it can be done.

Affliction is not a sickness; you can be afflicted and not sick, you can be sick and not afflicted or you can be both; but they are still different. Now if you fall into any of these categories the truth is that, although we lead normal human lives, the battle or the struggle we are fighting is on the spiritual level. Sometimes God allows the struggle so that we can awaken the spiritual man in us. It is to get us in a place where we have to rely solely on God. You see the very weapons we use while in our struggles are not human weapons but spiritual ones. In order to obtain total victory you have to use your spiritual weapons. Those weapons consist of prayer, positive thinking and believing that you are coming out of your situation. These tools are essential and powerful in the destruction of the enemy's strongholds. I challenge you to allow God to pull down every stronghold the enemy has placed or tries to place on you.

## II Corinthians 10:3-4
**3For though you walk in the flesh, we do not war after the flesh:**
**4(For the weapons of our warfare are not carnal, but mighty through God to the pulling down of strong holds;)**

It was now mid-August and George and I met with the surgeon to discuss the other test results. He reiterated what he had discussed a few weeks prior and mentioned once again his recommendation for me to have a Lumpectomy. He informed us that the surgery was scheduled for September 21, 2013. I was a little baffled because it was mid-August and I thought that the surgery would be scheduled sooner perhaps late August or early September. I once again made what appeared to be a negative situation turn into a positive outcome; it was no real sign of urgency and God needed more time to work on me and prepare me for what may arise ahead.

Let me interject here, I want you to always remember when you are in a bad situation try to see the good in it. There are countless stories I am quite sure you have heard where someone has missed a bus, train, plane, etc, and something went wrong and if they were on the bus, train, or plane they would have been injured and worst case scenario died. I am quite sure that person was upset when they missed the bus, train or plane because they wanted to make it to their destination on time. I know at some point and time they saw the good in what could have been a bad situation for them and counted it a blessing that they missed it. Learn to see the good and while doing so give thanks for the test. There is a reason why you are going through it in the first place. Just think if I would have given up, didn't believe that God can heal and did not see the good in my situation how would I have written this book to encourage you. I thank God for my test for without it I would have never stumbled across my strength; the strength to write this book for you.

**1 Thessalonians 5:18**
**In everything give thanks: for this is the**
**will of God in Christ Jesus concerning**
**you.**
**James 1:2-3**
**² My brethren, count it all joy when ye fall into**
**divers temptations;**
**³ Knowing this, that the trying of your faith**
**worketh patience.**

I waited patiently for the surgery date and in my wait I prayed constantly that the Lord would touch my body. I continued to encourage myself and feed myself God's Word; "by His stripes I am healed" I told myself daily.

**I Peter 2:24**
**Who his own self bare our sins in his own body**
**on the tree, that we, being dead to sins, should**
**live unto righteousness: by whose stripes ye**
**were healed.**

**The Surgery**
The surgery date was approaching and the night before the surgery, my good friends Elder Bouie and his wife Janean once again called and had prayer with me and the family. God truly blessed and I was encouraged. The next morning my Assistant Pastor, Bishop Charles Wright and his wife, Faye yet again called and had prayer with us, God once again blessed. I thank God for the prayers of the righteous for it truly availeth. Hallelujah! You may ask what do you mean Sharon by availeth? Merriam-Webster.com defines

availeth as to be useful or helpful to (someone or something); to be of use or advantage. Notice below the word, "much" at the end of verse 16, this word is an adverb describing a degree or amount. Webster uses "great in quantity, amount, degree, etc." to define it. Availeth much, then, gives a meaning of great use or advantage. So let's put it all together **The effectual fervent prayer of a righteous man availeth much** in essence means prayers offered with devotion by those who obey the Lord are able to produce a large quantity of benefit due to great power. Prayer is essential in our everyday lives, if we pray we produce a great deal of power; the power to deal with our everyday life situations.

### James 5:13-16

[13] **Is any among you afflicted? let him pray. Is any merry? let him sing psalms.**
[14] **Is any sick among you? let him call for the elders of the church; and let them pray over him, anointing him with oil in the name of the Lord:**
[15] **And the prayer of faith shall save the sick, and the Lord shall raise him up; and if he have committed sins, they shall be forgiven him.**
[16] **Confess your faults one to another, and pray one for another, that ye may be healed. The effectual fervent prayer of a righteous man availeth much.**

We are given so many reasons why we should pray some of which include suffering afflictions, sickness, confession of sins, the healing of the sick, forgiveness of sin; the list can go on and on. The verse that stands out is verse 13, the call for the elders of the church to pray, and yes they prayed. Thank God for the elders of the church. It is great to pray for ourselves but it is great to have backup!!

Let me continue on, it was a nice moderate day in September 2013. I went into surgery asking God to have His way in the surgery room and to bless the hands of the surgeon. While we waited in the waiting area for me to be called to be prepped for surgery, George whispered a prayer and shortly thereafter I was called. The prepping for the surgery was very intense and painful I had to constantly and quietly call on the name of Jesus. Because the tumor was slightly small, I had to have a small wire inserted into the breast so they can identify where to operate and to also check the lymph nodes in the surrounding area. God gave me the strength to endure it all. I remained calm and kept my composure. I can recall the technician saying you are handling this very well and he was very apologetic for any pain he was causing. I said to him "You have to do what you have to do and I have to do what I have to do". He smiled and uttered, "That's a good way to handle it". But my God, it did hurt! When the prepping was finally over I really had to exhale and give God praise for bringing me through the prepping process. My goodness I think the prepping process was worse than the actual surgery!!

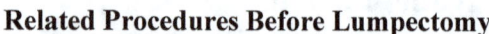

**Related Procedures Before Lumpectomy**
If your surgeon wants to check your lymph nodes during Your lumpectomy, you will need to have lymphoscintigraphy in preparation for a sentinel lymph node biopsy. And if your breast lump is too small to be

easily felt, a wire localization procedure may be done to help your surgeon locate and remove the lump.

Well, it was finally time for the surgery and as I was being wheeled into the surgery room I prayed all the way.

I recollect asking the surgeon can I pray for his hands and he replied most certainly. I asked God to bless the hands of the surgeon and the team in Jesus name. Amen.

The surgeon stated to me before he began the surgery, "Sharon everything is going to be alright" and off to sleep I went. "Mrs. Robinson. Mrs. Robinson you are in recovery"

3Breastcancer.about.com
I heard a voice say, as I opened my eyes it was the recovery nurse. I asked her where my husband was and she replied he was contacted and is on his way down to the recovery room. This surgery was different from the previous one although I was in pain I could move around a little better. When George arrived, he asked me how I was feeling although I was going in and out of sleep I responded I am in some pain but ok. He said thank you Jesus. Just then his telephone rang and it was my Assistant Pastor calling to check to see how I was doing. George responded she is ok but in pain, he responded let her know we are still praying. I thank God for the prayers of the righteous for again it availeth much.

The surgeon came into the recovery room and informed us that the surgery went very well. He stated that he had removed the tumor and that there was a tiny tumor on top of the existing tumor which they had to send for biopsy. He also informed us that he had removed several lymph nodes and sent them for biopsy to ascertain if the cancer had spread to the lymph nodes. He went on to say that as far as he could see the cancer had not spread. Thank God! He said as soon as he receives the pathology report which he would receive in a couple of days, he would let me know more in detail at my follow-up appointment the following week. At that moment I told God, "Anyway you bless me Lord I will be satisfied". I have too much work to do for the Lord and I must move forward and cannot allow the enemy to get into my mind and war against it. I must maintain the strength and faith that God had given me.

## 2 Kings 18:20
## Thou sayest, (but they are but vain words), I have counsel and strength for the war.

## Romans 7:23
## But I see another law in my members, warring against the law of my mind...

Whatever you are going through I urge you to not allow the enemy to place doubt, fear and negativity in your mind. Repeat God's word: **I have counsel and strength for the war.** God will give you the strength for the fight and the fight after that too! I know it all so well, God gave me the strength I needed to go through and while I was going through it, He gave me the strength to endure.

Not knowing what my next fight was going to be I kept my mind on God through prayer and continued to remain positive and did not allow any negative thoughts to overshadow me. Yes negative thoughts came and yes I heard negative stories, but I did not allow it to overtake me. The enemy tried his hardest to war against my mind, but I refused to allow him to take control of me or it. Why you may ask, because I TRUST GOD!!

**Psalm 28:7**

**The Lord is my strength and my shield; my heart trusted in him, and I am helped: therefore my heart greatly rejoiceth; and with my song will I praise him.**


**Isaiah 26:3**

**Thou wilt keep him in perfect peace, whose mind is stayed on thee: because he trusteth in thee.**

George and I met with Dr. Satterfield for my follow-up, and he reiterated what he had discussed with us after the surgery. He conveyed to us that the pathology report confirmed that the cancer had not spread and importantly had not spread to my lymph nodes; however, the second tumor taken was indeed cancerous and it was a different form of cancer. Well before he could go on I asked him what do you mean? He told me not to get too alarmed because the tumor was removed. He stated that the tumor had cells called HER2 which is a more aggressive form of cancer and if the cancer returned it would return aggressively. I said to myself, the devil is a liar; I curse that from of cancer form the root in the name of Jesus.

He stated that once I consult with the Oncologist they could better explain the cancer, its risk and what the best options for me would be. I told him that I was going to use my previous Oncologist who was already aware of what was going on and to please send her all the reports so that she could review them beforehand. He said "Mrs. Robinson don't worry" and I replied to "thank you".. I mentioned to him that I had a great support team and that I was going to get through this. He sat upright in his chair looked at me with great admiration and responded "You have the right attitude!" With God I knew that this sickness was not an affliction and was not unto death.

## John 11:4
**When Jesus heard that, he said, this sickness is not unto death, but for the glory of God, that the Son of God might be glorified thereby.**

I knew whatever the outcome was going to be God was going to be with me every step of the way. I was praying and hoping that I would not have to encounter chemotherapy or radiation. But I wanted to attend the appointment with an open mind and be receptive of what the doctor may say.

The following week George and I met with Dr. Fulman, my oncologist and she reviewed the pathology report and the pictures with us. She reiterated some of the things that the surgeon had already discussed. She expressed to us that the tumor was removed and that another tumor was found on top of the previous tumor and that particular tumor although smaller than the original tumor was cancerous as we already knew. She stated that if the cancer returned it would be more aggressive and could spread rapidly to your lungs, your brain, etc. I said to myself, the devil is a liar; I rebuke this right now and curse it from the root in the name of Jesus, it will not return. Have you ever planted a flower or a plant and sometimes the root of the flower dies for whatever reason whether it is too dry, overwatered, overheated, etc, it causes the plant to wither and die. I have had that happen to me on numerous occasions. Every now and then you have to take further action on your situation;

just like that plant whose roots have died you have to curse the very situation from the root to kill it. Are you familiar with the parable of the fig tree found in Mark 20 where Jesus cursed the fig tree? Why did He curse the fig tree? He cursed it because it was not bearing fruit; it was useless and deserved to be destroyed. At times our situations deserve to be destroyed and in order to destroy it completely it has to be cursed from the root. Therefore it cannot bring forth fruit. I had to curse cancer from the root. I asked God to kill every sign and every cell of cancer in the name of Jesus Christ. There is power in the name of Jesus.

## Mark 11:20
### And in the morning, as they passed by, they saw the fig tree dried up from the roots.

Dr. Fulman conveyed to us that I had Stage 1 cancer for the first tumor and that the second tumor was HER2 and in between Stage 1 and Stage 2. She assured me that it was it was detected early and removed. Thank God. Ladies I urge you to have yearly mammogram test; it can save your life. Never put off what you can do today by doing it tomorrow; today can make a huge difference and tomorrow may be too late.

### ıWhat is HER2/3 Cancer
HER3 is increasingly coming under investigation for its role in the development of cancer. This section of ResearchHERPathways.com focuses on the way HER3 may cause cancer cells to grow and spread in spite of currently available therapeutic agents, as well as its prognostic value and role in breast and ovarian cancers.

## What is HER2-positive breast cancer?

All cells have **HER2 receptors**, including healthy cells and cancer cells. In HER2-positive breast cancer, **tumor** cells have more HER2 receptors than normal. Too much HER2 makes these cancer cells grow and divide too rapidly.

### NONCANCEROUS CELL

HER2 receptor

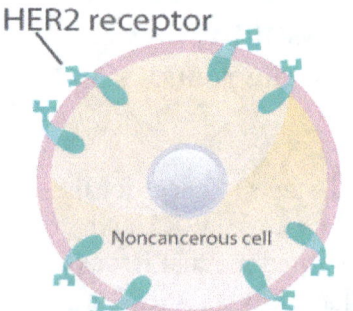

Noncancerous cell

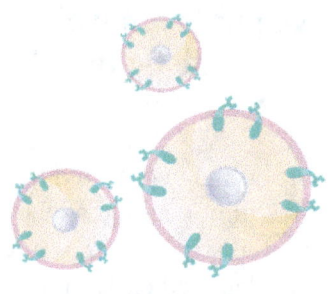

NORMAL AMOUNTS OF HER2 � RESULTS IN NORMAL CELL GROWTH AND DIVISION

**Cancer treatments called *HER2-targeted therapies* have been developed to target the HER2 receptor.**

Because of my diagnosis of the HER2 cell Dr. Fulman went on to explain what my options were. Out of her mouth came the words I surely did not want to hear, "I highly recommend chemotherapy followed by radiation treatments". I felt a lump in my throat and expressed a huge sigh. She explained to us that having the chemotherapy treatments as well as the radiation reduces the chances of the cancer returning and that it is a preventive measure as well. My heart was racing and at that moment I wanted to tell her I did not want the treatment because of all the stories I had heard about people who took chemotherapy. From what I had heard and read I knew that chemotherapy destroys good cells in your body and the doctor had confirmed that. She explained that the chemotherapy would be administered Intravenously (by infusion into a vein). She went on to explain the side effects of the chemotherapy. She explained that I could possibly lose all of my hair, may lose my eyelashes and eyebrows, she went on to say that my finger and toe nails may turn really dark, I may experience extreme fatigue, nausea, vomiting, constipation, diarrhea, headaches, peeling of hands and feet, sores in the mouth, loss of

Reference: 1perjeta.com

appetite, loss of taste, and brown spots. There was a small gleam of hope, she said it sounds bad but all will return back to normal after treatments are completed. Did I really want to do this I thought to myself? As I was sitting there listening to all of the side effects for a moment I thought-- maybe I should just believe God for my healing. As the oncologist began to discuss the four (4) options with me and my husband I listened attentively. I began to replace my negative thinking and feeling to a positive one. I thought to myself this is a good thing, if God brought me to this point He allowed it and therefore He was going to see me through it. So I began to consider the four (4) options which were given to me.

My husband and I discussed the options and we selected Option 2 which was divided into three phases, **Phase 1**: 12 weeks of treatment every two weeks = 4 times in those twelve weeks, **Phase 2**: 12 weeks of treatments once a week = 12 weeks treatment and **Phase 3**: For the remainder of the year, 2014 every 3 weeks for the duration of the year. She mentioned that during the chemotherapy treatments I would begin radiation in May, through July 2014. She went on to explain that the chemotherapy is long and hard but can be done. I was given a tour of the area where the blood would be drawn at each treatment as well as the area where I would have the chemotherapy administered. I was introduced to my nurse and was given my treatment start date. I strongly believe that this was the path I was supposed to take; I knew that God would be there with me and He would see me through the chemotherapy and the radiation process. I had learned from my previous colon cancer ordeal that whatever test I was faced with in order to move forward I had to face it; stand eyeball to eyeball to it and push forward. I will admit I was frightened of the unknown. I had to put it in my mind --that it did not matter how many people have died with what I had been diagnosed with or what happened to someone else in my situation, it had nothing to do with me and did not mean that the same thing would happen to me; same ordeal but different outcome. I could not focus on that, but had to focus on the one who gave me life and knows the very number of hairs on my head. I focused on Psalms 91:7 that although some may have fallen due to the illness it will not subdue me.

## Psalms 91:7
### A thousand may fall at your side, and ten thousand at your right hand; but it shall not come near you.

Sometimes we tend to allow what we see happen to someone else or have happened to someone else discourage us or dictate our outcome. This keeps you from maintaining your stand in faith. It doesn't matter how it looks and what you have heard **MAINTAIN YOUR STAND IN GOD** and your belief that all is going to be well! Whatever it is, it is not too hard for God. Jeremiah 32:27 asked a question, is there anything too hard for God? I will leave you to ponder what your answer will be. I encourage you while you are in your test; **stand** and watch God work on your behalf. You will then discover your answer.

## Jeremiah 32:27
## Behold, I am the Lord, the God of all flesh: Is there anything too hard for me?

I truly believed in my heart that God was going to get the glory out of my test. "No Test, No Testimony", I have heard this saying many times, but now I can truly attest to it.

I understood that my greatest challenge was ahead of me and I knew I had to accept it and face it in order to move forward. Trust me I did not want to endure the treatments, but it was before me and I had to do it so that I can put this chapter of my life behind me. I had to step out on faith and believe that God was going to see me through the treatments. You can't pray for rain and be afraid of the water. Fear and faith do not reside in the same vessel. Do not base your faith on your condition or situation, once you ask God to do something you have to believe that it will come to pass. I asked God for healing and I believe that it was going to come to pass. You have to believe even when you are not feeling your best. In the meantime until you have the physical manifestation of what is already yours in the spirit realm (according to your faith), you may experience some of the symptoms from the illness. Healing can come in various ways even through medication.

Medication can help you to deal with the symptoms and keep you from suffering so my advice to you is to take your mediation. I want to reiterate that God will see you through your situation if you allow Him too.

## 1 Peter 3:15
**But sanctify the Lord God in your hearts: and be ready always to give an answer to every man that asketh you a reason of the hope that is in you with meekness and fear:**

After George and I carefully chose what we thought would be the best form of chemotherapy treatment for me, my oncologist agreed with the option we selected. She stated that she was going to recommend the option we had chosen. This regimen was not as harsh as the other options but had to be taken for a longer period of time. I would rather have treatment for a longer period of time than to suffer badly for the next 3-6 months. Because I was still recuperating and healing from the surgery, my chemotherapy treatments were scheduled to begin the following month. While recuperating I continued to pray and ask God to take away all doubt and fear and continued to believe God for complete healing. I prayed that as I go through the chemotherapy treatments my body accept it and not reject it and while in the process not to allow me to look sickly and weak. I wanted to look as well and healthy as possible. The Word states in James 4:2 you have not because you ask not. I asked with certainty that I will receive that which I asked. Don't be afraid to ask.

## James 4:2
**Ye lust, and have not: ye kill, and desire to have, and cannot obtain: ye fight and war, yet ye have not, because ye ask not.**

# Endurance

Hebrews 12:1
Wherefore seeing we also are compassed about
with so great a cloud of witnesses, let us lay aside
every weight, and the sin which doth so easily
beset us, and let us run with patience the race that
is set before us…

# Chapter 3
## The Courage to Endure
## All for God's Glory

I began to anoint myself daily and continued to believe that God was going to get the glory out of all of this. I wanted to endure it all for God's glory.

## Phase One

The night before the chemotherapy treatment I once again prayed and believed God for complete healing during this process. Chemotherapy was all new to me; I must confess I was fearful of what was going to take place. Yes I know that fear and faith does not reside in the same vessel but it is human nature to be afraid of the unknown. I had to shake it off and prepare my mind for what was about to transpire.

It was late October and my husband and I began our usual routine by getting our sons, George and Chase ready for school. Once the boys were off to school, we rested a bit, had prayer and then prepared ourselves for my very first chemotherapy treatment.

### What is Chemotherapy

Chemotherapy is the use of anticancer drugs designed to slow or stop the growth of rapidly dividing cancer cells in the body. It may be used:

- As a primary treatment to destroy cancer cells
- Before another treatment to shrink a tumor
- After another treatment to destroy any remaining cancer cells
- To relieve symptoms of advanced cancer

The Oncologists being experienced in delivering targeted, individualized chemotherapy options while also proactively managing side effects.

**Chemotherapy delivery methods**
Some chemotherapy delivery methods include:
- Orally (by mouth as a pill or liquid)
- Intravenously (by infusion into a vein)
- Topically (as a cream on the skin)
- Injection
- Direct placement (via a lumbar puncture or device placed under the scalp)

When chemotherapy drugs travel through the bloodstream to reach cells throughout the body, it is called systemic chemotherapy. When chemotherapy drugs are directed to a specific area of the body, it is called regional chemotherapy.

As we approached the doctor's office, I had a clear head and I was ready to begin the chemo-therapy treatments. I was nervous but I knew I was going to get through it with the help of God. Before I went to consult with my oncologist my blood was drawn and vital signs were checked to determine if I would be able to have chemotherapy at the time. This is something that had to be done each time before all treatments. Once the blood work and vital signs are reviewed by the oncologist, you are then cleared or denied chemotherapy treatments. My oncologist checked my blood levels and blurted out "your blood levels are great you can proceed with treatment for the day". As I walked down the corridor the anticipation was high. My nerves began to get the best of me!! I began to tell myself these words: "I can do all things through Christ which strengthens me"; and "God did not bring me this far to leave me. This was my time to stand firm on God's word.

## Philippians 4:13
## I can do all things through Christ which strengtheneth me.

### Picture of Me Undergoing My Chemotherapy

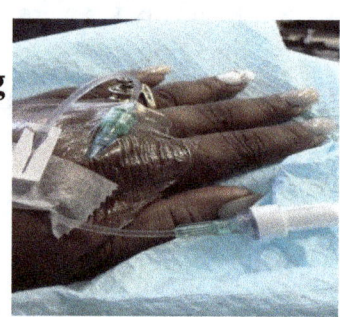

### Day 1 – Phase One

As George and I were walking to an available seat for treatment, an older gentleman and his wife who was receiving treatment were watching us. As I sat in the recliner, at that point the gentleman knew that I was the one who was going to receive treatment and in an orotund voice says, "Hey, why are you here, you do not belong here!" I was alarmed at first. After I placed my coat behind the seat I walked over to him and his wife and in a calm quiet voice said these words, "Although we are here, both your wife and I we are not here to take residence, we are only here temporarily; for this too shall pass". I stated to him that his wife was going to be alright. At that moment I took the focus off of me and placed it on him and his wife. He looked at me in dismay, paused for a moment and said "You know something you are right, I like you", "I like what you said". We conversed the whole time they were there and every chance I was given I encouraged him and his wife. Before they left he said that I encouraged them so much and he thanked me for the words of encouragement.

I felt so pleased that I was able to encourage someone even though I was going through myself.

By this time, a nurse came over to us singing "Hello Mrs. Robinson, it's you Mrs. Robinson".... and introduced herself as my nurse who will be administering the chemotherapy. I smiled. She said I know you must hear that song all the time and I said, "yes I do". We chuckled. She blurted out we have a "Newbie" here. I was wondering why she said that and later on it hit me, was it said perhaps because I was the only one in my area that had my hair while others around me did not. She explained the chemotherapy process and said that treatments were going to be administered intravenously. She then began the prepping process and shortly thereafter the chemotherapy treatments were administered. As the treatments were flowing into my veins I prayed and asked God to get me through all of the treatments and not allow my body to reject the medication, but allow the medication to do what it was suppose to do for me.

## Psalms 91:10
## There shall no evil befall thee, neither shall any plague come nigh thy dwelling.

As I was taking the treatment a young woman sitting across from us kept starring at us. Why is she staring over here so much I wondered? Shortly thereafter she comes over to where I was sitting. She said I know you were probably wondering why I was staring so hard. She went on to say that she was contemplating if she should come over. She began to share her story and experiences with my husband and I of how she had breast cancer some years ago and the tumor was as big as a tangerine and her doctor told her that she would need a mastectomy. She told the doctor when it was her time to leave this world she would be leaving with both of her girls (her breasts) that God had given her. I smirked. She mentioned to us that she prayed to God and asked Him to heal her and although she asked for healing she was going to follow her doctor's instructions because her healing can come through the medication. She added that she had surgery to remove the cancerous tumor and she received chemotherapy and radiation and to date was cancer free at least breast cancer free. Wow look at God if he can do it for her he can do it for me. Going back to what I stated previously you have to be positive and believe that God can heal; you can't live a positive life with a negative mind. She disclosed to us that she had bone cancer and she knew in her heart that God was going to see her through it the same way He'd seen her through her breast cancer. At the time she was undergoing chemotherapy treatments and having bone marrows every three (3) months. She said with such authority, "This too shall pass". I listened to her amazing story as she confirmed some things I had stated. God knows how to get your attention and let you know that all will be well. I began to share my story with her and I encouraged her like she encouraged me. I said to her that with God we were going to be alright. I asked her if I can say a word of prayer with her and she replied yes and we silently prayed with her. There is a lesson to be learned in all instances of our lives and God can use anyone at any given time to encourage and enlighten you. I am guilty of judging others based upon their appearance and shun away. I am quite sure you are guilty of this too! I must admit I was a little skeptical of this young lady because of her appearance and loudness but she was an inspiration to me.

My first day of treatment was very interesting it was a long day, a bit tough and somewhat painful process. I really didn't have much time to focus on me most of the time was spent talking to the various people around me who were there for some form of treatment. I thank God that He gave me the strength to endure my first treatment. I felt weak and tired but I made it through bearing in mind one down and many more treatments to go.

## Day 2 – Phase One

My second treatment was an experience as well. My good friend and sister, Charlene accompanied me to the treatment to relieve George. This was her first time seeing how chemotherapy was done. The poking and blood work was a venture within itself but you do get an opportunity to meet a lot of interesting people along the way. A young man was sitting next to me and he was really sick, he was very apologetic because he was regurgitating. I told him that I understand that he was not feeling well but better days were ahead. I wanted to speak a positive word to him in case he was feeling down. I asked him if I could say a word of prayer with him and he responded yes. I quietly prayed and asked God to bless him and help him to endure whatever treatment he was undergoing without getting too sick and to give him strength in Jesus name Amen. His face had lit up after the prayer and he turned to me and said, "Thank you sister I needed that prayer, thank you so much, God bless you sister". I noticed that he had stopped regurgitating and was able to fall asleep shortly thereafter.

I continued to uphold him in prayer as I sat there. As I sat there canvassing the area I observed a young woman in the bed across from us sobbing. She was all alone and seemed to be in a lot of pain. I could not get to her at that moment but felt compelled to see her before I left. Upon leaving I went over to her and asked her if I could have a word of prayer with her and she said yes, I gently placed my hand on her leg and asked God to touch her body in Jesus name.

She was so thankful. This was totally out of my element I had never done anything like this before. It is such a good feeling when you are able to encourage others and give them hope beyond what they can see. Sometimes a simple prayer can go a long way and put someone on the path of believing that God can heal them or put them in the path of positive thinking.

I began to really believe that this was God's divine will for me and I was supposed to be at this site to uplift and encourage and importantly for God to be glorified. Again this was totally out of my element, normally if I would see someone that needed prayer, I would pray for them silently; never in a million years would I ask them if I could pray with them.

In my observation I have found that many people are looking for that little glimpse of hope. We have to come out of our element to give that someone the hope that they so desperately need. We may not always understand God's plan but at some point you will. We are placed in situations so that we can go to the next level or the next chapter in our lives. We are all on assignment whether you believe it or not. In blessing others we are blessed. You have to be bold enough to allow God to use you. Use me Lord!! Glory be to God! Through my praying and encouraging those around me I too felt uplifted. If you can forget about your situation for a moment and pray for the person next to you your strength and faith will be increased and will prepare you for your next encounter. I dare you to stop what you are doing now and encourage the person next to you. You never know what someone is going through and that simple prayer can make a big difference. It could be the difference between life and death you never know. I have had several experiences where I looked at a person on the train and began to pray for them. I can recall a time when I prayed for an individual on the train and the next day as they were talking to their friend I heard them say that they had a situation the day before and that they could not believe how everything worked out for them. God used me to pray for that person and they were blessed. Prayer does work!

## 2 Corinthians 9:14
## And by their prayer for you, which long after you for the exceeding grace of God in you.

I recall Charlene telling me that she was totally impressed how I was allowing God to use me. She pointed out that I had encouraged her during the time she was there. That's what it's all about. We spend too much time worrying and not enough time encouraging.

### A Prayer for You
*Lord I ask right now that you bless the person reading this right now. Father God I ask that you would give them the strength to endure and grow in faith. Give them the boldness to not only pray for themselves but to pray for the person right next to them, across from them and that person who is not even in their view. As they pray for that individual encourage them too and give them the courage to move past their test. For it is written that you will not let us be tested beyond what we can bear; and that when we are tested you will provide a way of escape. Thank you for the way of escape. In Jesus name. Amen.*

As I was approaching my third round of chemotherapy, although I was not feeling my 100% best I was thankful that I was enduring the treatments. Every day I would look in the mirror and to my surprise I still had a head full of hair and for that I was so grateful. I was holding on to a little glimmer of hope that perhaps I would not lose my hair.  Late one night when I awoke out of my sleep I realized that my head wrap was loosely moving around.  I stumbled into the bathroom to see exactly what was going on and when I removed the head wrap I discovered that some of my hair was in the head wrap.  I took my hand and gently ran it across my head.  Literally within minutes I was completely bald.  I couldn't believe it!!  I stood in the mirror looking in disbelief.  Although my oncologist prepared me for this I refused to believe that it was going to happen to me.  I stood there for about ten minutes looking at all my hair in the sink and began to cry.  I admit I was upset.  After I got over the initial shock of being completely bald I looked at myself in the mirror and said these words, "I am fearfully and wonderfully made".  Psalms 139:14 I will praise thee; for I am fearfully and wonderfully made: marvelous are thy works…. God created each one of us, in a wonderful way. God made us the way we are and for a specific purpose. When we understand that, then we can have peace that whatever ailments or perceived problems we have in life God ordained them. At times when you feel like God is far from you, comfort yourself, God is ever present and aware of your problems and needs.  If He bought you to it He will see you through it.

### Psalm 139:14
**I will praise thee; for I am fearfully and wonderfully made: marvelous are thy works; and that my soul knoweth right well.**

Although the human side of me was upset, I had to remind myself that losing my hair was temporary and my hair would grow back permanently.  I had to focus on the outcome not what the human eye could actually see at the moment.

**II Corinthians 4:18**
**While we look not at the things which are seen,**
**but at the things which are not seen: for the**
**things which are seen are temporal; but the**
**things which are not seen are eternal.**

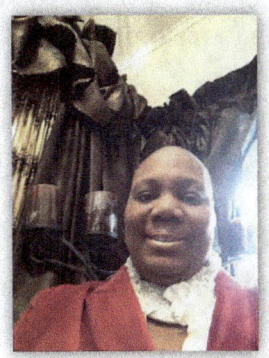

I must admit losing my hair was a humbling experience. I loved my hair and losing it so quickly was devastating. Every strand of my hair was gone, I was completely bald. I began to examine my current situation and tried to see the good in what I thought was a bad situation. I thought to myself, I am clean from the top down; I was cleansed so that I could be made new again. Hallelujah! When you really think about the word clean you think of being cleansed from dirt, stains, or marks, free from contamination or disease. What are you saying Sharon, the point I am trying to make is that sometimes we have to be cleansed and in doing so we are made new again. How many times have you had a bad cold or the flu and the doctor tells you to let it run its course. Once the cold or flu has run its course it is cleansed from your system and therefore when it is over, you feel like a new person. We need to be cleansed from time to time.

## Leviticus 13:40
**A man who has lost his hair and is bald is clean.**

I had to come to the realization that although I was bald I was in the cleansing process; And while in the process I was going to be made new, stronger, wiser and steadfast in God. God was going to restore all that was lost!

## 1 Peter 5:10
**And the God of all grace, who called you to his eternal glory in Christ, after you have suffered a little while, will himself restore you and make you strong, firm and steadfast.**

Once I accepted the fact that I was bald I embraced it and wigs became my best friend! When I attended my treatments I wore shorter styles because I did not want to offend anyone or make anyone feel down. I always wanted to cut my hair into a short style but was always afraid so I took advantage of the new me for now. I looked at it this way too, at least now I did not have to be concerned with sitting in the beautician half the day. That was a good thing!! There is always a blessing in everything, like I mentioned earlier in the previous chapter, you have to pull out the good in what may appear to be a bad situation. Looking for the good in a bad situation is good for you, it gives you hope and keeps you focused on the positive. The word says in

## Philippians 4:8
**Finally, brethren, whatsoever things are true, whatsoever things are honest, whatsoever things are just, whatsoever things are pure,**

**whatsoever things are lovely, whatsoever things are of good report; if there be any virtue, and if there be any praise, think on these things.**

I must say 2013 had been a trying year for me and my family. Have you heard the saying when it rains it pours, well it was pouring in my life. One Friday evening I was looking at my eldest son, George Cameron and noticed that the right side of his face seemed a little twisted. I asked him was he feeling okay and he said that the right side of his face was feeling numb. I automatically thought that it was Bell's palsy; I called the pediatrician immediately. When the doctor returned my call, I explained to him my son's condition and before I could continue, he said it sounds like he may have Bell's palsy and he wanted to see him immediately. I forgot all about my condition, I felt like my whole world was crumbling. Now a condition was on my child, I felt helpless. I could deal with me but not the condition on my child; it was unbearable. I let George sleep with me so that I could watch him; I took the blessed oil which my pastor prayed over and while my son slept I anointed him and prayed over him. Out of nowhere I began to cry uncontrollably. I did not want to disturb him while he slept. As I sat there watching him he awoke looked up at me and asked, "Mom are you crying?" I said in a quiet voice "Yes I am". He looked at me hugged me and said these words, "Mom we are fighters, we are going to be fine, you'll see, God is with us". I said to him in a shaking voice, "You know something you are so right, we are fighters". God will not put more on you than you can bear. Although while you are going through it may be painful and hard, you must realize that God is working it out for you. Through your sufferings and pain you are being made a stronger and better person. Clearly God was up to something in my life, I couldn't possibly be going through all of this for nothing. In Romans 8:18 we find that Christians will likely face difficult life situations and therefore should not be surprised when God sometimes takes what is perfect and subjects it to a humble status so that a greater good might be accomplished. We must grab a hold to hope! This stage of suffering I was enduring was merely a transitional period; a transitional period from groaning to glory. Hallelujah. I believed God for my son's healing; this was another test to keep me praying, keep me believing and above all keep me strong.

## Romans 8:18
## For I reckon that the sufferings of this present time are not worthy to be compared with the glory which shall be revealed in us.

### ₁What is Bell's Palsy
Bell's Palsy is the paralysis or severe weakness of the nerve that controls the facial muscles on
the side of the face – the facial nerve or seventh cranial nerve. Patients typically find they suddenly cannot control their facial muscles, usually on one side.

A person might have Bell's palsy first thing in the morning - they wake up and find that one side of the face does not move. If an eyelid is affected, blinking might be difficult. Bell's Palsy usually starts suddenly. Bell's palsy must not be confused with cerebral palsy, a completely different condition.

Most people who suddenly experience symptoms think they are having a stroke. However, if the weakness or paralysis only affects the face it is more likely to be Bell's palsy. Approximately 40,000 Americans develop Bell's palsy each year. The National Health Service (NHS), UK, reports that about 25 to 35 people out of every 100,000 develop Bell's palsy each year. It is classed as a relatively rare condition. It more commonly affects people over 15 and under 60 years of age, and affects men and women equally. Bell's palsy can last anywhere from 3 months to a year depending on the case.

I continued to anoint my son each night and upheld him in prayer. I constantly spoke with him and encouraged him. Each day he seemed a tad bit better. In the face of dealing with my son's situation; I continued to undergo my chemotherapy treatments. The treatments were becoming more intense and I was feeling more fatigue and sick. There were times when I did not want to go but I had no choice if I wanted to put it behind me so that it could benefit me in the end. God had really helped me thus far and I had to continue. My oncologist stated that I was doing very well with the treatments. She went on to say that she was impressed with me as a patient and how I carried myself and how encouraging I would be during the course of my treatments. She expressed to me that she uses me as her prime example telling other patients about how encouraging and inspiring one of her patients were during treatment. She indicated that my frame of mind was incredible. I was delighted to hear her say that! I was elated to be used as an example to let someone see that you don't have to look like what you have or currently going through. With God's help you can get through whatever it is.

I want to encourage anyone who might be expecting to have or currently having chemotherapy, radiation, or may be scheduled for any form of surgery be sure to obtain all of the help you need; be sure to attend all scheduled appointments and attend every treatment for as long as the doctor advises. If you plan to have surgery undertake the attitude of expectancy that God is going to see you through it. Not only expect that all is going to be well but believe it. I urge you to follow the doctors' regimen as well as pray and read God's word for strength. I am reminded of the story of Shadrach, Meshach, and Abed-nego. These men worshipped God and had a strong belief in God. They refused to bow down to the golden image (god) that the King Nebuchadnezzar had built. Because of their disobedience to the King they were thrown into an immense, blazing furnace. The flames were so hot that it killed the men who escorted them into this furnace. These three (3) men went into the furnace with the expectancy that God was going to be with them and see them through. They stood strong in their belief that God was going to deliver them. They did not stagger or alter their belief they stood tall and firm. Sometimes as Christians or people in general when the tough gets going we tend to bend and alter our way of thinking. But we must stand firm on what we believe no matter how it looks. God was indeed with Shadrach, Meshach, and Abed-nego when King Nebuchadnezzar looked into the furnace he saw four (4) people walking in the midst of the furance and not the three (3) men he originally had placed there.

King Nebuchadnezzar marveled that the men emerged from the furnace unharmed, with not even a hair on their heads singed or smell of smoke were on their clothing. He had to admit that the fourth person looked like the son of God and not the golden image (god) he had built. God always has a way to get our attention. If God can be with Shadrach, Meshach, and Abed-nego and not allow them to be burnt, imagine what He can do for you.

1Reference: Medialnewstoday.com

You may be in the fiery furnace of life, but remember you are in it for a little while and the fire will not touch you.

You are coming out without being burnt just like Shadrach, Meshach, and Abed-nego. I say again you will not look like what you have been through if you just trust God. You are welcomed to read Daniel chapter three in its entirety to get the full story of Shadrach, Meshach, and Abed-nego.

I was moving right along, I had approached Phase 1 with that same attitude of expectancy that God was with me and was going to see me through it as I discussed previously. During the course of Phase I God did not allow me to experience all of the side effects however I did experience the extreme fatigue; I had no idea that being fatigued can make you feel so sick. I felt sick, nauseated and weak; I experienced numbness in my toes, my nails turned extremely dark and loss of hair. God did not let me lose my appetite but I did lose my taste buds, food was not enjoyable but I forced myself to eat for strength. I continued to take my vitamin C, B6, B12, D and a multi-vitamin. Through it all I can say that God truly blessed me; it could have been much worse. I MADE IT!!! Hallelujah!

## Phase Two
I was now onto Phase 2, I had to gear my mind and get ready to face whatever was to come with the second form of treatment. Although this treatment was not supposed to be as severe as Phase 1 I could still experience the extreme fatigue, nausea and weakness. I went into Phase 2 with the same mindset as Phase 2. I continued to believe that God was going to restore my health.

## Jeremiah 30:17
## For I will restore health to you and heal you of your wounds, says the Lord....

During this ordeal I had to reach a point in my life where I really believed God and hand to stand on His Word. Not that I didn't before, but I was in a situation where I had to really put my confidence in what I believed. I began to read God's Word with more compassion and understanding. God knows how to get you where He wants you to be. I began to see things differently and clearly. My praise was different, my worship was different and my outlook on life was different. I wanted more of God because I knew He was the only one who can heal, set free and deliver me. I established a praise that only God can give. As a Born again Christian have you ever been at home or in your car and you begin to think on the goodness of God and what He got you out of and you just break out in a "Just Because Praise". Yes I was there, I would break out in a "Just Because Praise", Just because I knew that God was able, Just because God was good, Just because God was going to see me through.......My God "Just Because God is God".

There were times when I did not feel my 100% self but I did not want my inability to attend church at the time to interfere with my husband's ministry at our church. I wanted him to continue working in the capacity that he was working because he needed to be as close to normalcy as possible. He also needed to continue to do the work of God although I could not. My husband was a trooper, he had to go through all of this with me, be my support, take care of the responsibilities at home especially on those days when I could not, attend football games as well as take care of his obligations at our church (attending meetings, etc.) and with God's help he did all of this without murmuring or complaining. George fulfilled his obligations like nothing was going on. Not unless it was a dire need I dare not ask him to stay with me at home but gave him the freedom to fulfill his duties at home, work and at church. I wanted God's blessings to come on me and overtake me again and again without any interference from me. Deuteronomy 28:1-14 became so relevant. I needed God to bless the fruit of my body by healing me of cancer. And I took the scripture to heart, **And all these blessings shall come on thee and overtake thee**.

## Deuteronomy 28:2
**And all these blessings shall come on thee, and overtake thee, if thou shalt hearken unto the voice of the LORD thy God.**

My pastor always read the blessing plan found in Deuteronomy 28:1-14, it had been a scripture he spoke of for many years. It was not until now that this scripture really manifested in my life. This chapter is a very large exposition of two words, the blessing and the curse. They are real things and have real effects. If you read this chapter you will find that blessings are written before the curses. God is slow to anger, but swift to show mercy. God loves to bless his people and takes delight in doing so. Blessings are promised based upon the condition that we hearken unto the voice of God. You can't expect His blessings if you interfere with His plan. I prefer the blessings and not the curses.

# Deuteronomy 28:1-14

And it shall come to pass, if thou shalt hearken
diligently unto the voice of the LORD thy God,
to observe and to do all his commandments
which I command thee this day, that
the LORD thy God will set thee on high above all
nations of the earth: ² And all these blessings
shall come on thee, and overtake thee, if thou
shalt hearken unto the voice of the LORD thy
God. ³ Blessed shalt thou be in the city, and
blessed shalt thou be in the field. ⁴ Blessed shall
be the fruit of thy body, and the fruit of thy
ground, and the fruit of thy cattle, the increase
of thy kine, and the flocks of thy sheep.
⁵ Blessed shall be thy basket and thy store.
⁶ Blessed shalt thou be when thou comest in, and
blessed shalt thou be when thou goest out.
⁷ The LORD shall cause thine enemies that rise
up against thee to be smitten before thy face:
they shall come out against thee one way, and
flee before thee seven ways. ⁸ The LORD shall
command the blessing upon thee in thy
storehouses, and in all that thou settest thine
hand unto; and he shall bless thee in the land
which the LORD thy God giveth thee.
⁹ The LORD shall establish thee an holy people
unto himself, as he hath sworn unto thee, if thou

shalt keep the commandments of the LORD thy God, and walk in his ways. [10] And all people of the earth shall see that thou art called by the name of the LORD; and they shall be afraid of thee. [11] And the LORD shall make thee plenteous in goods, in the fruit of thy body, and in the fruit of thy cattle, and in the fruit of thy ground, in the land which the LORD sware unto thy fathers to give thee. [12] The LORD shall open unto thee his good treasure, the heaven to give the rain unto thy land in his season, and to bless all the work of thine hand: and thou shalt lend unto many nations, and thou shalt not borrow.

[13] And the LORD shall make thee the head, and not the tail; and thou shalt be above only, and thou shalt not be beneath; if that thou hearken unto the commandments of the LORD thy God, which I command thee this day, to observe and to do them: [14] And thou shalt not go aside from any of the words which I command thee this day, to the right hand, or to the left, to go after other gods to serve them.

## Phase Two - Day 1

It was day 1 of Phase 2 treatment. As we approached the facility I went in with the expectation that God was going to bless me and enable me to endure this treatment as he did in Phase 1. I went in repeating Philippians 4:13, I can do all things through Christ which strengthens me.

As George and I entered the treatment room to look for a seat, I scanned the room as I always did and began to pray for all the patients who were receiving different forms of treatment. I asked the Lord to continue to restore health not only for me but to all in the room. As I sat in my seat I noticed a couple sitting across from us that I had never seen before, the gentleman was in a lot of pain and it seemed as though they could not administer treatment and was waiting to hear from the doctor if it was okay. I wanted all my treatments to be administered the day it is supposed to be and not have it postponed because my vital signs and/or blood levels were either too high or too low. So I knew if I felt that way this gentleman probably felt the same way. I began to pray for him and asked the Lord to bless him to receive treatment and to help his pain to subside. A few moments later the gentleman's doctor came over and asked him a couple of questions, the doctor then gave approval for his treatment to be administered. I began to thank God for that in my seat. I know within my heart that I was not only there for myself but for others.

The administering nurse came over to where George and I were sitting and reiterated what the oncologist had already discussed regarding Phase 2 of treatment. She explained what it entailed, the side effects as well as the medication I was about to receive. She elucidated that I would be monitored for the first fifteen minutes of treatment to ensure that I would not have an allergic reaction to the medication. She stated that along with treatment I would be administered Benadryl. Phase 2 was already different than Phase 1, I had begun experiencing a burning pain during the very last phase of treatment and remained calm during the pain, but it was not easy. Just as I prayed for the gentleman across from me I had to pray for myself that the pain would subside. The pain at times was excruciating but I took it without complaining. I would tell myself "this too shall pass; it will all be over after a while". We have to sometimes speak positivity into our lives in order to gain some sort of sanity. I know you are probably saying talk to yourself that's insane! No it's not insane you have to sometimes encourage yourself. You will find that you can comfort you. It works!

My treatments seemed to come so quickly, it seemed as soon I was done with one treatment it was time for another. Being an only child I didn't want to bother my mom so much although I knew it wasn't a bother at all. It is really good when you have family and friends who will step in and fill the gap when you need them too and assist wherever they can as well as relieve my mother, mother-in-love and husband when needed. George had been so good at coming with me to my treatments but he needed a break from time to time. I thank God for my family and good friends who were there for me. My good friend Janean who I call my little sister accompanied me to my treatment to relieve my husband so that he could go to work. I followed the same routine like any other day when I entered the treatment area I would always speak to everyone in the surrounding area. As I addressed those around me I recall one of the patients who I would see and speak too would never say anything but would always stare. This particular day which so happened to be the day my friend/sister was with me after saying my good mornings to everyone I began to take off my coat and I felt the curtain move. Just as I sat down I heard a quiet voice say excuse me and I turned to see who was speaking to me and guess who it was? It was the patient who had never said anything to me. I began my conversation with her by saying good morning and asked her how she was feeling and she responded to me in a whisper, I have been watching you every time you come for treatment. She went on to say that I was always cheerful, bubbly and how amazing I looked each time she would see me. She then said something that really encouraged me; she said that I was such an inspiration to her and that seeing me each time gave her hope. I was simply ecstatic at her remark. I thank God for allowing me to be an encouragement to others and I am thankful that my light was shining for her to see. The way you carry yourself and your mannerism can have a great impact on a person. I thanked her so much for sharing that with me.

## Matthew 5:16
## In the same way, let your light shine before others, that they may see your good deeds and glorify your Father in heaven.

During the course of treatment I was advised by Dr. Fulman, my oncologist that I should see a genetic counselor to determine if my sons were at risk to inherit breast cancer and or colon cancer. I met with a genetic counselor, Carol Rung and was tested, thank God all tests came back negative. Hallelujah. I encourage you if you have been diagnosed with cancer and any other disease to see a genetic counselor especially if you have children. You want to ensure that your children are healthy or if something is detected early they can be seen and helped early on.

### ıWhat Does a Genetics Counselor Do?
A genetics counselor is a professional who helps people make decisions based upon genetic information. For example, prospective parents might consult a genetics counselor in order to determine if they want to find out

whether their potential offspring might be at risk for being born with an inherited disorder. Genetics counselors also help people determine if they want to know their own risk of developing a genetic disease such as heart disease and breast cancer.

Genetics counselors also work alongside other health care professionals including doctors, geneticists, nurses and social workers. The goal is to help individuals and families make informed decisions about their health and to assist clients in finding the services that best serve their needs.

## Phase 2 Treatment

During one of my treatments I was speaking with a young woman who was undergoing chemotherapy for breast cancer; she was complaining about the treatment and how she had lost all of her hair. She asked me how I dealt with the loss of my hair. I shared with her my initial shock and devastation of losing my hair and after getting over the shock I had to come to the realization that it's only hair and that being bald was temporary not permanent. I told her to try to see the good in her situation and that her test was only given to make her strong. I expressed to her not to dwell on the negative aspect of the medication but to concentrate on the fact that it is given to make her feel better. I asked her if she wanted to get better and she replied, "Why certainly". I responded to her that if she wanted to get better she had to think the way she responded, "Why certainly I will be better". I told her she had to constantly remind herself each day that she will get better and her hair will grow back. This is a temporary test not a permanent test, I uttered to her. At first she looked at me crazy and said nothing, she belted out, "Wow you are so positive, I need to talk to you every time I see you, I needed to hear that". The same words I had told her were the same words I told myself over and over again; it was my reinforcement.

I was counting down the time, it was February 28th and I had two more treatments of Phase 2 to go and I was excited. I began Phase 2 with great expectation that God was going to bring me through it. I met with Dr. Fulman as I always did, we went over my blood work and vital signs and I was cleared for treatment. She informed me that they were conducting a clinical investigation and because of my diagnosis of breast cancer I met the criteria to participate in the study. She asked me if I would be interested in participating in the study as she explained the purpose of the study that it may aid in the development of new diagnostic test kits and devices for particular diseases and illnesses. All I would need to do was give blood. She explained that a sample of my blood will be stored and used for future research purposes; she also indicated that my blood samples may be used for genetic research. I was totally interested in participating in the clinical investigation especially if it is going to help someone else. I filled out the consent form with great excitement. I thank God for allowing me to be able to help someone else.

## Hebrews 2:18
### Because he himself suffered when he was tempted, he is able to help those who are being tempted.

We all have had some form of suffering and have been tempted to give up but somehow we made it through our storm.

Reference:1About.com

Sometimes we are placed in a storm so that we can be a blessing to someone else. Don't be afraid to share your story.

In the midst of Phase 2 God was healing my son. Every day I would see his face trying to return to normalcy. Although the process was long I continued to pray with him and believed that God was going to make him whole again. As I lay sleeping one Saturday morning my son ran into the room yelling with great excitement, "Mom look at me, look at me". With great anticipation I looked at him and his face was approximately 95% normal. As aforementioned when you have Bell's palsy, you cannot control the side of your face affected by it. He was able to close both eyes together tightly at the same time before he was unable to do that, his right eye was tearing on its own without having to use artificial tear drops and his smile or laugh was beginning to return to normal. You could not tell that the right side of his face was ever twisted although when the Bell's palsy was in full swing you really could not tell that my son had it unless he smiled or laughed or when he spoke certain words. I began to praise God for his healing and his complete healing. It was a long road, but God was fulfilling his promise to me. I cannot express enough that praying works and believing God works. God is so good!! Hallelujah! Once God has begun a work in you, he will complete it. He has to finish what He has started.

## Philippians 1:6
**Being confident of this very thing, that he which hath begun a good work in you will perform it until the day of Jesus Christ:**

## My Last Treatment of Phase 2

It was the last day of Phase 2 treatment and I awoke with praise in my mouth and a dance in my feet. Why are you praising God and dancing for you may ask!! Well let me tell you Phase 1 and 2 were the hardest treatments to go through and God had allowed me to go through it without ever missing a treatment. Yes it was not easy but I made it. There were days I felt so sick and my body ached so badly I could hardly move. But I took it and when asked how I was feeling I would always respond "good". Your words have power; the power of the tongue can speak life or death to your situation,

## Proverbs 18:21

## Death and life are in the power of the tongue: and they that love it shall eat the fruit thereof.

As I entered the oncologist office I entered with great excitement knowing that I was getting closer to completing my treatments. Dr. Fulman, my oncologist came into the examining room with a smile on her face, "Today is graduation day for you, you made it" she uttered. She proceeded to give me a hug. I said "Thank God I made it". I smirked and asked where my cap and gown. We laughed. She then asked "Was it fire and brimstones as many people make it out to be" and I said to her "Well let me put it this way, I was in the fire but God did not allow the flames to overtake me. "I felt some heat but God held back the flames". She looked at me in astonishment and said, "You are truly an inspiration and such a true trooper". My vital signs and blood work were good and I was cleared for my last treatment of Phase 2. Hallelujah!! The oncologist told me that soon after the last treatment of Phase 2 I would begin to see my finger and toenails return to its normal color and the nail pain would go completely away in a couple of weeks, my body aches would subside and the burn marks would begin to clear up.

I was well ready for some form of normalcy. Although I was extremely fatigue I felt good. She stated that when I begin Phase 3 I would not experience some of the things I had previously experienced but will continue to be fatigue but it would become less. I was so glad to hear that! Things were looking up. I was looking forward to returning to church and working more days on my job. My treatments would be scheduled for every three weeks as oppose to every week so I welcomed the change. I was waiting to hear when my radiation treatments would begin.

As I entered the treatment area I was jubilant, I got my favorite seat and although my regular nurse was not there I still felt good. After my treatment was completed I felt like a million bucks! Some of my ailments had already begun to clear up. I began to see hair particles which meant my hair was beginning to grow back.

During the course of Phase 2 of treatment I recall times when my legs, arms and hands felt like heavy lead, I could barely lift my legs but I tried not to let it stop me and even managed to go to work even in pain. I had to do it and not allow the pain to consume my mind and cause me to give in to the pain. I thank God for supportive co-workers who assisted and helped me. There were other times when I was in excruciating pain and I laid in my bed in tears, moaning and praying quietly trying not to disturb my husband. It was those times when I called on Jesus to ease the pain. I prayed and cried myself to sleep and when I awoke in the morning although the pain was there it was more bearable. It was a long rocky road but I made it. For whatever reason the last three treatments seemed to be the hardest and I started to experience more pain than usual. Parts of my body developed what appeared to be burn marks but I took it in stride knowing that this too shall pass. I continued to take my vitamins and placed coco butter on the marks and went on my merry way.

One of my co-workers who had experienced what I was going through asked me how my finger and toe nails were and asked did I lose any. I told her that so far, so good, my nails were in tack.
She began to share her story about how her finger and toenails came off when she was having the treatment. Although bewildered I was glad she shared that with me. God has a way of preparing you for what is about to come. A week later my toe and fingernails began to hurt so badly. I examined my nails closely and noticed that two (2) of my nails seemed to be a little loose and my hands and feet were extremely dry and peeling. I placed band aids on the nails that were loose so that they would not fall completely off. I immediately called my oncologist and mentioned it to her, she informed me that it was a normal occurrence and told me to soak my hands and feet in hot salt water and baking soda and use poly bacitracin cream on my nails so that they would not get infected. I am grateful that my co-worker informed me of this beforehand because had I not been prepared I would have panicked. Touch your neighbor and say "preparation!" I rejoice in preparation!!

## II Chronicles 29:36
**And Hezekiah rejoiced, and all the people, that God had prepared the people: for the thing was done suddenly.**

All I want to be is a vessel of honor for God and fit for the master's use. I want to be able to encourage and inspire those around me and all those who I may come in contact with. I want to be a blessing to you the reader and want to encourage you that you can make it. God had to purge me from head to toe to get me to where I am today. I have grown more rooted in God and in His word than I would have ever imagined.

## II Timothy 2:21
**If a man therefore purge himself from these, he shall be a vessel unto honour, sanctified, and meet for the master's use, and prepared unto every good work.**

## New Beginnings
It hard been a long journey; it was Friday March 21, 2014, spring had sprung and I was on my way to work and not treatment. I had been attending treatments every Friday for the last few months and oh what a great feeling it was not to attend treatment. It was a sign of a new beginning for me. When one beginning reaches its end, it is time for a new beginning. There are many new beginnings, new job, new friends, new relationships, new house; new car the list can go on and on. But there is nothing like a new beginning from a past struggle to a present **VICTORY**. You have a new outlook on life when you actually make it through the struggle.

## Isaiah 43:19
**Behold, I will do a new thing; now it shall spring forth; shall ye not know it? I will even make a way in the wilderness, and rivers in the desert.**

It was a blessing to be able to finally go to work two Fridays consecutively. Sometimes we take little things for granted, just to be able to get up on your own, move around on your own, lift your legs on your own, able to travel to your destinations on your own, etc, is a blessing. We are not doing it on our own it is God who allowed us to wake up with breath in our body and enables us to do so many things on our own. We need not take nothng for granted, but should wake up with a thankful heart and begin to thank God each day for the little things. Don't assume that you are doing things of your own efforts, although the alarm clock helped wake you up, remember it was God who allowed your ears to hear the alarm.

## Ephesians 5:20
## Giving thanks always for all things unto God and the Father in the name of our Lord Jesus Christ;

As I have been mentioning throughout the course of this book; we often times have struggles and during those times we need to be thankful for the struggle and grateful for life. I know it is easier said than done but if you begin to practice being thankful in the struggle it will become second nature. While I was in my struggle although hard at times, I gave God thanks regardless of how I was feeling. I encourage you to give Him thanks and watch God work, try not to complain but try to smile through the pain. That is what kept me from day to day while undergoing my treatments. It was not me; it was God who kept me while in the struggle. I have the utmost faith in you that you too can make it through your struggle. I will touch and agree with you right now that whatever the struggle you are in you will make it in Jesus name. You are coming out!!! Take that and run with it!

## Phase 3 of Treatment

By the time my first treatment of Phase 3 came around, April 4th to be exact, I was feeling better than I had felt in a long time. I walked into the treatment center with a little more pep in my step. Things were looking up for me. My oncologist was not there and I was seen by another doctor who stated that she was happy to see that I had completed Phase 2 of treatment and doing well. She checked my blood work, cleared me for treatment and I was on my way to begin Phase 3 of treatment. I went into the treatment area with high expectations that I was going to get through Phase 3 with God's help. If I could make it through the harshest of treatment I was going to be alright!!! The treatment time was not as long as the previous treatments. The nurse informed me that the treatments would become a little less after the initial Phase 3 treatment. My treatment went well although I still felt fatigued and nauseous but still I felt good. God is good, He knows our infirmities and although He was tempted like we are, yet He was without sin. Sometimes the struggle causes a person to give up on God and to give in to the temptation, but we cannot allow the temptation to overtake us, we must move forward with a positive attitude. I know I keep stressing to you to believe that God can heal you, that God can help you through your struggle, to move forward while in your struggle, having a positive attitude and not giving up, but I must keep writing it so that it is embedded into your spirit while reading about my experiences.

**Hebrews 4:15**
**For we have not an high priest which cannot be touched with the feeling of our infirmities; but was in all points tempted like as we are, yet without sin.**

## Phase 3 of Treatment

It was my second treatment of Phase 3 and I was feeling good and remaining positive. I thank God every day for a positive attitude which was also affecting those who I came in contact with. While at my second treatment I saw a young lady whom I hadn't seen in a while and I was very happy to see her. I often thought about her and I prayed for her daily. She introduced me to her mother who had accompanied her to treatment. She said to her mom, this is the young woman I was telling you about, she is such an inspiration to me, always smiling, encouraging and always looking great! I was extremely touched by her comment. Although I am going through this situation, while on my journey, I want to be able to encourage and uplift someone else who is traveling in this path. I feel that in this journey my mission was to encourage and uplift.

We exchanged telephone numbers so that we could keep in contact with each other. I asked her how she was doing and she said, "Not so good" I said, "No, you are doing well". I began to explain to her that sometimes our body may be saying one thing but our lips should say the complete opposite. If our body is feeling bad we must speak positive to the situation. We have the power to speak those things as though they are. She gave me a blank stare. She began to tell me how she could not eat and that she lost so much weight. I can tell she was feeling really down.

But you are alive and that's what counts, I uttered. Remember all of this is temporary, you will gain your weight back and you will be feeling like your old self again, I said to her. I did something out of the ordinary, I asked her to repeat these words with me, "I am fearfully and wonderfully made, I am going to be fine, as she repeated the words I said now that you have said it your assignment is to believe it. She smiled and leaned over to her mother and said, "You see I told you she was inspiring". Before I went to my seat for my treatment I looked at her once again and said "You are going to be what", and she said, "I am going to be fine". I said to her to speak it into existence. Continue to pray and things are going to begin to look up for you; you'll see I uttered. She said yes, we will pray for each other.

I want to say to you the reader, things are going to look up for you too. It doesn't matter what your struggle is or how long you were in the struggle, you are going to be fine! Now say it with me, "I am going to be fine", I am blessed". *Lord at this moment I ask that you would bless the person reading this, I ask that you would intervene in their situation right now. You are a God that cannot fail, you can do all things, you can heal, you can set free, you can deliver, right now God do it. Help the person reading this to believe in you and what you can do. Lord heal the hurt, mend the broken heart and give them the strength, the courage, the desire to go on and not look back in the name of Jesus. Amen.*

Two weeks had passed and I received a text from the beautiful young lady I had mentioned in the previous paragraph and she wrote, "I am eating a little more and I started back cooking a few days ago. Tell me if you have the energy to write your book", she wrote, "I know it's hard but we gain a bit of energy and strength daily". She went on to say "Thank you for your prayers and continual words of encouragement, your words have gotten me through a lot of things". I thank God that she seemed to be doing a little better from our last conversation. God is good! I wrote her back and informed her that I was glad to hear that she was doing better, and that things were looking up. I told her to continue to keep a positive attitude and that we were going to get through this. Sometimes I am amazed at God and how He used lil ol' me so that He can be glorified. Hallelujah!

## Matthew 5:16
**Let your light so shine before men, that they may see your good works, and glorify your Father which is in heaven.**

## And Thus My Journey Continues……..
My journey continues and I had to follow the path in which it took me. My oncologist informed me that for precautious reasons she wanted me to undergo radiation therapy. I was not surprised because she had mentioned it prior to my beginning chemotherapy treatments. Before I go on I want to explain what radiation is and how it works.

### 2What is Radiation Therapy
Radiation therapy also called radiotherapy is a highly targeted and highly effective way to destroy cancer cells in the breast that may stick around after surgery. Radiation can reduce the risk of breast cancer recurrence about 70%. Despite what many people fear, radiation therapy is relatively easy to tolerate and its side effects are limited to the treated area. Your radiation treatments will be overseen by a radiation oncologist, a cancer doctor who specializes in radiation therapy.

## How Radiation Works

Radiation therapy uses a special kind of high-energy beam to damage cancer cells. (Other types of energy beams include light and x-rays.) These high-energy beams, which are invisible to the human eye, damage a cell's DNA, the material that cells use to divide. Over time, the radiation damages cells that are in the path of its beam normal cells as well as cancer cells. But radiation affects cancer cells more than normal cells. Cancer cells are very busy growing and multiplying 2 activities that can be slowed or stopped by radiation damage. And because cancer cells are less organized than healthy cells, it's harder for them to repair the damage done by radiation. So cancer cells are more easily destroyed by radiation, while healthy, normal cells are better able to repair themselves and survive the treatment.

There are two different ways to deliver radiation to the tissues to be treated: a machine called a linear accelerator that delivers radiation from outside the body pellets, or seeds, of material that give off radiation beams from inside the body Tissues to be treated might include the breast area, lymph nodes, or another part of the body.

## Why Radiation is Necessary

Radiation is an important and often necessary form of anti-cancer therapy because it is able to reduce the risk of recurrence after surgery. Although it's quite possible that your surgeon removed all the cancer, breast cancer surgery cannot guarantee that every last cancer cell has been removed from your body. Individual cancer cells are too small to be felt or seen during surgery or detected by testing. Any cells that remain after surgery can grow and eventually form a new lump or show up as an abnormality on a test such as a mammogram. Research has shown that people who are treated with radiation after lumpectomy are more likely to live longer, and remain cancer-free longer, than those who don't get radiation. In one large study, women who didn't get radiation after lumpectomy were shown to have a 60% greater risk of the cancer coming back in the same breast. Other research has shown that even women with very small cancers (1 centimeter or smaller) benefit from radiation after lumpectomy.

**Radiation Treatment.....The Beginning**
I visited the Farber Center for Radiation Oncology located in Manhattan and fell in love with the facility and staff. The staff was amazing; they cared a great deal for their patients and were very helpful. What impressed me the most was the cleanliness of the facility and the fact that the staff knew each patient by their first name. Dr. Leonard Farber was great; he sat and explained the radiation treatment how it worked and went on to explain in his words what would NOT happen while having radiation treatments. He joked and stated that I would not glow in the dark, I would not beep at the airport and importantly I would not experience any pain during treatment. He informed me that the treatments were going to be five days a week for approximately eight weeks. I will admit that when I was told of the duration of the treatments I was a little taken back. I had no idea that the radiation treatments would last so long especially since I was having chemotherapy treatments as well. Dr. Farber went on to say that the biggest joy he receives is seeing his patients walk in one way and upon the completion of the treatment leaving almost their full selves again. As Dr. Farber continued to speak I was preparing myself mentally, I was saying to myself chemotherapy and radiation go hand and hand, just do it!

2Reference: breastcancer.org; about.com

Thank God the doctor and staff who made me feel comfortable. I felt good and confident that I was in good hands. Once again I knew that God was with me and this was just another test for my testimony.

## Luke 21:13
## And it shall turn to you for a testimony.

After meeting with Dr. Farber I met with the supervisor who prepped me for the radiation treatments. She explained what exactly was going to take place and thus the prepping process began. I was what was called "tattooed" for the radiation treatments and ready for treatment a few days later.

### 3What Are Radiation Tattoos?
Before having breast radiation, you may need to have skin markings or radiation tattoos put on your breast skin. These marks help your radiation therapist accurately aim the radiation at your treatment area. You may be having five days or six weeks of radiation, and every treatment should be aimed at the same place in order to prevent recurrence and spare healthy tissue. It's a bit like using a bulls-eye target for archery, darts, or rifle practice -- having a clear target area to aim at improves results.

### Blue Tattoos For Treatment Safety
Radiation tattoos will be blue or black, and will be created using a drop of ink and a very slender needle. You might feel the needle stick, which should hurt no more than a mosquito bite. These tattoos won't wash off, so you will be able to shower or swim anytime during treatment without losing these important markings. However, if a skin marker is used instead of a permanent tattoo, be careful to keep these marks dry until the end of treatment. Your breast

radiation tattoos will be tiny -- about the size of a freckle, or 1 millimeter. There will be at least four tattooed dots, each marking one corner of the area to be radiated. Having these skin marks in place helps to speed setup for each treatment as well as increases the safety and accuracy of your radiation. Radiation tattoos will be created during your treatment simulation, before treatments begin.

**Marks of Survival**
Your radiation tattoos will be permanent, and serve as a reminder that you are a breast cancer survivor. These tattoos also provide a visual reference for other doctors who may need to know where you received radiation.

My first few days at the Farber Center were great; again I felt that I was in good hands as I moved forward in the healing process. God had given me such a peace and I wanted to continue to move forward in the process and continued to thank God for total victory.

Upon writing what tattooed meant and seeing the words: "Marks of Survival" I felt chills go through my body. I began to think about how Jesus died on the cross for you and me and how he bore the signs on his body, the hole in his hands and feet and the markings on his head due to the thorns being placed there. God suffered for us and he never said a mumbling word. God had marks of survival on Him for you and for me. What a mighty and courageous God who died for us so that we can live. As I lay on the examining table to begin my first day of radiation therapy, the radiation therapist stated that the tattoo markings are in place and that the radiation will be aimed at that particular tattooed area.

3Reference: breastcancer.org; about.com

I was then positioned on the table in the angle I was to lay at every session and the radiation therapy treatment began.

As I lay still and quiet I began to pray and ask God to continue to dry up any and all cancer cells and to dry it up from the root and cut the branch so that it will **NEVER** return again anywhere in my body.  I rebuked the powers of sickness.

**Luke 17:6**
**And the Lord said, If ye had faith as a grain of mustard seed, ye might say unto this sycamore tree, Be thou plucked up by the root, and be thou planted in the sea; and it should obey you.**

**Job 18:16**
**His roots shall be dried up beneath, and above shall his branch be cut off.**

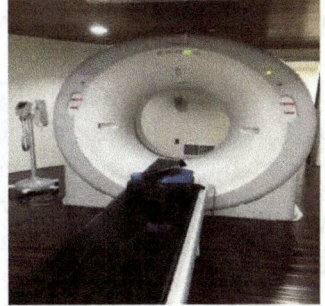

**Picture of the Examining Table for My Radiation Therapy**

As I lay there I thought about the tattoos that were placed permanently in my body and pondered to myself, girl you have the marks of survival, **"I AM A SURVIVOR"** not once but twice.  Hallelujah!  Because of God and God using the doctors I am truly a SURVIVOR and I have the

marks to prove it. My God, my God! I am led to write this to whomever is reading this right now; no matter what you are going through you are coming out and you too will bear the marks of survival. It's ok to cry and it's ok to go through. You are stronger and you are wiser. I ran across a saying that was so relevant and it read: **"I am Thankful For My Struggle, Because Without It, I Would Not Have Stumbled Across My Strength".**
This statement is so true you have power to determine where your strength lies. You are much stronger than you think, so go through my sister, my brother, you are coming out with more strength than you can ever imagine. Hallelujah!

While undergoing radiation therapy I was still undergoing Phase 3 of treatment. Phase 3 of treatment was scheduled to continue until December 2014. As I entered the treatment area a nurse uttered that I always come to treatment happy, bubbly and looking good all the time, she asked me a question, "How do you do it"? Have you ever broken down and cried because of the situation, she asked. I replied, "Yes I am human and I can say that yes I broke down on numerous occasions but it took one good time where I cried like a baby". Once I got it all out of my system, I wiped the tears from my eyes and told myself that I shall live and not die, I have to live for my family, my family needs me. I mentioned to her that whatever situation a person is going through that it is good to cry and let it out, it helps in the healing process and makes you feel a little better. I went on to say that once you have that really good cry, not allow the situation to overtake you, you overtake it. She said, "Wow your strength is amazing". I said to her it is not all me but its God who grants me the strength. I will write it over and over again, you will gain strength in your situation, God has equipped all of us for the battles of life and with the strength to endure, you have to dig deep within your being and be determined to rise above your situation.

## Psalm 18:39
**For thou hast girded me with strength unto the battle: thou hast subdued under me those that rose up against me.**

## Psalm 19:14
**Let the words of my mouth, and the meditation of my heart, be acceptable in thy sight, O LORD, my strength, and my redeemer.**

It is ironic that the nurse asked me the question--if I had ever broken down because of my situation. I guess it was lingering in my sub-conscious mind. One day while undergoing one of my radiation treatments I began to feel overwhelmed and my emotions got the best of me. Before I knew it the feeling had overtaken me and I felt as if I had enough; enough radiation, enough chemotherapy, tests, poking, blood taking, needles and fatigue. In the heat of the moment and with tears in my eyes, I began to think about the what ifs, what if the cancer comes back, what if the chemotherapy doesn't work, and what if I am doing all of this in vain, what if I die. I wanted to throw in the towel but as I lay there I began to think about how far I have come. Would God want me to throw in the towel now? I had to speak to myself, I had to be like David in I Samuel 30:6 and encourage myself. How many of you can relate to that? Life is a journey but sometimes the journey takes unexpected detours. And this was my unexpected detour. Never in a million years would I think that I would be diagnosed with cancer let alone twice in the same year and undergoing chemotherapy and radiation treatments.

## 1 Samuel 30:6
**And David was greatly distressed...... but David encouraged himself in the Lord his God.**

I had to speak life to myself and to my circumstance fast and in a hurry! I could not allow these feelings to succumb me. I had to shake it off! It was not the time to throw in the towel, not the time to give up or give in, not the time to stop running but to stay on course so that I could obtain the prize. Why is it that when you are almost at the finish-line you want to give up? I was almost at the finish line, and I had to keep running, and not look back for victory was coming I told myself as the tears streamed down my face. Hallelujah!!!! Glory!!!! I felt God's presence and anointing.

## 1 Corinthians 9:24
**Know ye not that they which run in a race run all, but one receiveth the prize? So run, that ye may obtain.**

### Running the Race
As I lay there I imagined myself running an actual race, I saw myself at the start-up line I was in position, chin up and waiting for the whistle to blow. I imagined the world watching and anxious to see me run. I was not thinking at the moment about the prize but concentrating on completing the run. The whistle is blown and I take off with enormous speed. During the course of the race I lost my footage and almost slipped. For a moment I wanted to give up, but I couldn't I was getting close to the finish line, I had to get back on track, gear my mind and run, run, run.

I continue to run although the finish line was not in my view but I knew it was ahead. I start to feel weak, but I run, I start to feel tired, but I run. I can do it I tell myself!! With God **I can do all things through Christ which strengtheneth me**. **(Philippians 4:13)** I am gaining ground so I must endure to the end so I continue to run. Victory is coming!!!

## Hebrews 12:1
**Wherefore seeing we also are compassed about with so great a cloud of witnesses, let us lay aside every weight, and the sin which doth so easily beset us, and let us run with patience the race that is set before us,**

## II Corinthians 12:9
**And he said unto me, My grace is sufficient for thee: for my strength is made perfect in weakness. Most gladly therefore will I rather glory in my infirmities, that the power of Christ may rest upon me.**

So to you I say "Run, Run, Run, you may not see the finish line in your view but stay in the race; you are almost there, don't give up". Patience my sister, patience my brother!! Your victory is closer than you think. Your strength is made perfect in weakness, you are gaining your strength back; you are gaining momentum. Keep on running!!

**Headed Toward the Finish Line – I Can Finally See the Finish Line**
Following my overwhelming episode, I attended the next session of radiation treatment feeling alright. The doctor

informed me that I had completed the first phase of treatment and now onto Phase two of treatment. He explicated that I had ten more days of treatment. Wow, I uttered to myself; I was getting close to completing my treatments. The finish line was closer than I thought. He went on to say that in Phase 1 the entire breast was treated and in phase 2 the area in which the cancer was located will be treated. The radiation treatments will also be shorter he added. I was very happy to hear the news and it could not come at a better time! I began a countdown to the finish line. Nine, eight, seven, six, five more days I continued towards the finish line. The closer I got, the more excited I would get. Four more days and wouldn't you know it I received a call from the doctor's office stating that the radiation machine was getting repaired and therefore I would not be able to have radiation treatment. Awww, so close….. I was so looking forward to putting this treatment behind me and having three more to go, but I was determined not to let it get me down, I continued the run. Three, two, I could see the finish line and finally one more day of radiation treatment. With sweat running down my face, my heart beating fast and with great anticipation I crossed the finish line. My last radiation treatment was completed and I was giving God all the praise for bringing me through. Thank God I made it!

While undergoing radiation the area being treated turned extremely dark and began to peel. I would periodically experience a shooting pain around the perimeter. It was not an unbearable pain but an annoying pain that lasted only for a few moments. I learned to persevere through the pain. I am thankful that the treatments were not hard and God had placed me in the right place and in the right hands. During the course of treatment I walked many times in the heat, I met a young woman who worked near my job and was undergoing treatment as well at the center and she allowed me to travel with her as a guest on Access-A-Ride. The days I rode with her were extremely hot and I did not have to walk in the heat. God always seem to open doors for me.

The time had come and I had finally reached the last day of radiation treatment. It was a bittersweet moment for me because I had gotten use to the routine of going to radiation treatment every day and besides the staff was so compassionate, nice and caring. Yes I would miss them and I thank God for the experience but my time there was up. I had reached the finish line of that particular race and had accomplished what I sat out to do. Getting to the finish line was long and I had a meltdown but I didn't give up, I made it. I felt like I wanted to throw in the towel but I did not, I used the towel to wipe my tears and I made it! Thank God I made it!!!

Shortly after my radiation treatments were completed; my skin began to return to its original color. Although I was not feeling my 100% self I felt good and well on my way to feeling my 100% self again. I want to take this moment to write how much I love God and all that He has done in my life thus far. I don't know how I would have made it without God on my side and the prayers of family, saints and friends. I know that God allowed me to go through this for a reason. I want to write this to someone who is having a hard time believing that God is real. I want to tell you that yes God is real, prayers are real and healing is real. I can firmly say without a shadow of doubt in my mind that if you believe in Him you can receive an abundance of blessings. I want you to experience the same joy and peace that I have obtained from God. Even in the midst of your circumstance you can obtain peace that surpasses all understanding. Many times we go through circumstances that we don't know how we are going to get out of but I want you to know that you can come out of any circumstance. You must believe that God can bring you out. Being diagnosed with cancer two times in the same year I could have lost my mind, but God, He kept my mind and gave me joy and peace in the midst of my circumstance. It was not always easy but I believed that God was going to bring me out and I kept a positive attitude. I encourage you to believe it, receive it and watch God work in your life.

## Romans 15:13
**May the God of hope fill you with all joy and peace in believing, so that by the power of the Holy Spirit you may abound in hope.**

## Philippians 4:7
**And the peace of God, which passeth all understanding, shall keep your hearts and minds through Christ Jesus.**

### Another Round of Chemotherapy
Three weeks had passed and it was time once again for treatment. I was excited to report to the doctor that my radiation treatments were completed. I felt good and I felt blessed. As I entered the treatment area I scanned the area for my favorite seat and it was available. As I sat down a young woman entered and sat in the seat adjacent to me and we began to talk to one another. She shared her testimony with me that this was her second battle with cancer and that she was diagnosed with cancer two years ago and how God bought her out the first time. She went on to say that when she was diagnosed the first time she

placed it in God's hand and let Him work it out for her. She said she prayed and believed God then and she believed God now. I sat there and listened to her story; I felt even more uplifted and encouraged knowing that I too had been diagnosed with cancer two times. I begin to share my testimony with her, as I was speaking she interjected and said God is going to bless us again. She stated to me to continue to believe God and keep it in God's hand. We surely encouraged each other. As I was getting ready to leave she grabbed my hand and echoed these words: "May all the blessings of God be upon you, your family and your friends Amen. "I receive that in Jesus name". God knows when you need encouragement.

**A Testimony of Victory**
I have to report victory for a co-worker who shared her testimony with me and it is well worth sharing. It is amazing to me at times to see what God can do and how He works. Before I go on I have to lift my hands and give God the praise. Both of us were diagnosed with breast cancer, she was in Stage 4 and because of the position of the cancerous tumor it was inoperable. To try and shrink the tumor her doctor wanted her to begin chemotherapy intravenously however her body rejected the treatment. The next step was for her to take the chemo pill and have an extensive radiation treatment. During her ordeal whenever we would see each another we would always have encouraging words to say regardless of how we were feeling. I would always ask her how she was doing and her response would always be I am doing well. We both always had a positive attitude and tried not to allow negativity into our spirit. We would both thank God together for our healing. As I was going to lunch this particular day she began sharing her testimony with me in an exciting voice she said "I have a victory report". I was eager to hear the victory report. She went on to express to

me how she is done with her chemotherapy treatment and that the tumor was shrinking.  She said as her doctor was telling her the exciting news she literally dropped to her knees in the office and began to thank God all the while her doctor was telling her to please get up.  She went on to say that the doctor didn't understand not only was the cancer shrinking but had shrunk in an unimaginable amount of time.  When God does a mighty work He does it so the world can see who He is and what He can do.   At Stage 4 she should have been in the hospital but her continual prayers and belief that God was going to heal her gave her the strength to go on.    She expressed how weak she became at times but she persevered and received the strength she needed to go on.

## II Corinthians 12:9
**And he said unto me, My grace is sufficient for thee: for my strength is made perfect in weakness. Most gladly therefore will I rather glory in my infirmities, that the power of Christ may rest upon me.**

As she was speaking my heart was overwhelmed and I felt blessed that our paths had crossed.   She was a real encouragement to me.  I share her story and wrote this book to encourage and inspire you.   I pray that what I have written thus far has given you the faith, strength and the courage to endure your test.  You too can be an overcomer.

### My Sister's Keeper – A Word of Encouragement
A few weeks later I saw a co-worker who I had not seen for quite some time. I began to share briefly what I had been going through.  As I shared my story she began to cry.  I began to encourage her and told her I was alright; that God was good and He was seeing me through.  I spoke about

how God had been blessing me as I was undergoing chemotherapy treatments. She said "My God you are so strong". She began to tell me about one of her friends who had currently been diagnosed with colon cancer and how discouraged he was. I informed her that I was in the midst of writing a book and that I wanted to give her and her friend some encouraging words from it. She was thrilled. When I returned to my desk I wrote her these words:

Going through Colon Cancer and Breast Cancer all in the same year (2014) and having to encounter chemotherapy and radiation was a challenging experience. At the time I could not understand why I was chosen to go through this test however I began to be thankful for the struggle. I realized that without the struggle I would have never stumbled across my strength. I encouraged him that what he was going through was temporary and was set up for permanent victory. I went on to write, If you change your mind-set you can change your situation. The key formula to healing/victory is: **Prayer + Visualizing the Answer to your Prayer + Praise + Positive Attitude + Forgiveness = VICTORY** which in time gives healing.

- Prayer – Equip yourselves (Matthew 21:22) Explained in Visualize your answered prayer
- Visualize – Visualize the Answer to your prayers – Prayer is the God-given tool to strengthen your faith and Trust in God.; (Matthew 21:22)
- Praise – Praise your way to victory – On a daily basis give God praise for what He can and will do.
- Positive Attitude – Do not allow negativity into your spirit; try to keep a positive attitude and keep positive people around you.
- Forgiveness – This is a hard one. So many times people have done things that hurt us. Forgiveness is giving up your right to hurt someone that hurt you. It is impossible to live on this earth without getting hurt, offended, misunderstood, lied to, lied on and/or rejected.

Such is life. We need to get over it; I know it's hard but in order to obtain complete victory we have to let some things go. It might be easier said than done but we can do it, you can do it. Let's do it together!!!!

I went on to write, be encouraged you are coming out of your current situation. You will be set free, you will be delivered, you will be healed saith the Lord. Go in peace my friend. I am praying for you! She called me and with a trembling voice she said the words were so comforting to her and she really needed to read that.

## Time Waits For No One
Two months had passed since I had completed my thirty-eight sessions of radiation and although I was experiencing some minor discomfort I felt good. I was continuing my chemotherapy treatments and taking it in stride. Time was approaching for me to have a mammography and I continued to thank God for complete victory. Although I was nervous I still believed that there was nothing too hard for God so I continued in faith as I did every day.

## Examining Day
It was a Saturday morning and I began to prepare myself mentally and spiritually for my mammogram. Although a little nervous I walked into the office at ease and calm. I believed that God did not bring me this far to leave me and I believed that He was going to give me the victory.

**1 Corinthians 15:57**
**But thanks be to God, which giveth us**
**the victory through our Lord Jesus Christ.**

As I sat and waited to be called I began to reminisce about the different healings that God had performed in the Bible. I reflected on Peter's mother-in-law, she was sick with fever and Jesus just touched her hand and the fever left from her body (Matthew 8:14-17), all it took was just a touch, I thought about the lepered man went to Jesus and asked Him to make him clean, Jesus put forth his hand and touched him saying "be thou clean" and immediately his leprosy was cleansed (Matthew 8:2-3), Jesus made the blind to see, the lame to walk (Matthew 15:29-31) my God he even raised Lazarus from the dead (John 11). If God can heal, set free and deliver them He sure can heal cancer. Let me ask you this question: Is there anything too hard for God? I leave you to ponder on it!

Before testing began; I asked the technician will I be able to get the results of the mammogram the same day. She informed me that once a person is diagnosed with breast cancer, mammogram results are given the same day so they are not left wondering and worried. What a relief!!
I was happy to hear that although I was seeing my doctor in a week, but a week can be a long time when you are waiting on results. Your mind plays tricks and the devil would have toyed with my mind until I'd seen her. As I begin the testing I prayed silently as I continued to believe God for my healing. Every time a picture was taken I began to thank God for what He had done in my body. Once the mammogram was completed I had a seat in the waiting area so that the doctor could review the pictures. As I sat there waiting I was nervous, I had to encourage myself again and again. The wait seemed so long, it was approximately thirty-five minutes, the technician returned and informed me that she needed to take several more pictures. Of course my mind began to race. I asked her if everything was ok? She said more pictures were needed to determine if what was seen was scar tissue or if the cancer

had spread although he was certain that it was scar tissue. As she took the pictures I began to pray again and speak life and not death to my current situation. Once she was done I went back into the waiting area and there I continued to pray. My nerves were shot and my hands sweaty!!! As I sat there the devil was surely on his post, my mind was racing. I had to detour my mind and do exactly what the bible says to do in **Philippians 4:8 Finally, brethren, whatsoever things are true, whatsoever things are honest, whatsoever things are just, whatsoever things are pure, whatsoever things are lovely, whatsoever things are of good report; If there be any virtue, and if there be any praise, think of these things.** I thought to myself if God can raise Lazarus from the dead He is well capable of healing cancer. I rebuked every negative thought and tried to remain positive. The doctor walked over and handed me a piece of paper which contained my results. I glanced down at the paper with one eye open and one eye closed. Once I saw the results I didn't know if I should cry or laugh. I implied to the doctor that I had read the results but all of the hell I have been through, all of the chemotherapy and radiation treatments, I wanted to hear her tell me my results. She looked at me in disbelief, I totally understand" she replied. She smiled and said "Mrs. Robinson, you are cancer free and a copy of the pictures and the report will be sent to your doctor". I cannot begin to share with you how relieved, overjoyed and most of all thankful I was. As I walked out of the office towards the elevator, the tears poured down my face and I had to utter a thank you Jesus out loud. God for my healer, He did it again for me!! I could be added to the list of those God had healed; I could be placed in between the woman with the issue of blood who God had healed and the woman who had fever and God touched her and the fever immediately left her body. My God, he had touched me again!! I was cancer free for the second time. Even as I write this section my eyes are filled with tears thinking on the goodness of God and all He had done for me. I am ever so grateful for what God has done a second time. I was so happy to be able to inform my family and close friends about another chapter in my life where God has proven Himself to be a healer. I was excited to share the good news! I took a picture of the results with my phone and shared it with my husband and mother. Oh the joy that came to me when I knew that I was free, when my savior found me, put his arms around me , oh the joy that came to me rung out in my head.

God is able to do all things but fail. Once again I want to encourage you to go the doctor, get checked; early detection is always the best detection. If I had waited and decided not to go the doctor at that time or not go to the doctor at all, I may not have been able to write this book today. Do it my sister, do it my brother, it may save your life.

**Still in the Race…..Four More Treatments to Go……**
When I saw my oncologist the following week, she reviewed my report from the mammogram and congratulated me on being cancer free. It was great to hear those words come out of her mouth. It was music to my ears. My treatments were narrowing down, four more to go, time is moving and my feet were running. I am still in the race, running toward the finish line. I considered myself blessed to able to do the chemotherapy treatments and my body not reject it. While in the race I was weary, I was worn but I continued. I could hear the words in I **Corinthians 9:24** in my ear, "Run All". I had to run all to obtain the prize at the end.

**I Corinthians 9:24**
**Know ye not that they which run in a race run**
**all, but one receiveth the prize?**
**So run, that ye may obtain.**

### An Unforeseen Obstacle

Why is it that when you are close to victory obstacles always seem to occur? I was running with patience the path that was set before me and up ahead was an unforeseen obstacle. With four more treatments left and cleared to have my treatment my oncologist advises me that my Carcinoembryonic Antigen (CEA) level was slightly elevated and she wanted to re-do the blood work and schedule a colonoscopy to ensure that the colon cancer had not returned or to ensure that nothing unusual was going on with the colon.

### What is a Carcinoembryonic Antigen (CEA) You Ask

A carcinoembryonic antigen (CEA) test is a blood test used to help diagnose and manage certain types of cancers, especially cancer of the colon. The test measures the amount of CEA present in the blood. If you already have cancer, this test helps a doctor determine if the treatment for the cancer is working.

An antigen is a harmful substance that is released by cancerous tumors. If you are receiving treatment or have had surgery for a previously diagnosed cancer, a higher amount of CEA in your body suggests that the cancer has not gone away. It may also mean that cancer has spread to other parts of the body. Smoking increases the amount of CEA in your body. You should tell your doctor if you smoke.

#### 4When Will Your Doctor Order the Test?

A doctor might order a CEA test for the following reasons: To help diagnose cancer in someone whose symptoms suggest that cancer is a possibility, To find out if the treatment a patient is receiving for their cancer is working. The treatment might include surgery, chemotherapy, or radiation, or a combination of all three to find out if a cancer has come back (recurred) later on.

A CEA test is most useful to monitor patients who already have been diagnosed with a type of cancer that is known to produce CEA. Not all cancers produce CEA. Increased levels of CEA may be found in the following cancers: colorectal (colon) cancer, medullary thyroid carcinoma, breast cancer, cancer of the gastrointestinal tract, liver cancer, lung cancer, ovarian cancer, pancreatic cancer, prostate cancers, Importantly, the CEA test is not useful in diagnosing or screening the general population for cancers. It should not be used to screen or diagnose healthy asymptomatic people, even people at high risk of cancer. If you are diagnosed with cancer, your doctor may begin monitoring levels of CEA before you begin treatment to establish a baseline amount. A single CEA value is usually not as informative as gathering many values over a period of time. Your doctor will perform the test repeatedly before, during, and after treatment to assess changes over time.

When the doctor informed me of the information I was totally caught off guard. I was not expecting to hear this especially after hearing the good news of being cancer free. I asked her what all of this means. I have been told that I am cancer free and now something may be going on with my colon again. I was baffled. She expressed that it could very well mean nothing because my levels were not extremely high but she wanted to take precaution and re-do the blood work for reassurance. I advised her that it was time for me to schedule my colonoscopy anyway and she told me to try and schedule it immediately. While I was undergoing chemotherapy I called my gastroenterologist to schedule an emergency colonoscopy only to find out that my gastroenterologist was no longer at the facility where I originally had my first colonoscopy and the facility had since moved. Sometimes you have to look at the big picture and see how things play out in your life. As I reflected on the past, the gastroenterologist was no longer at the facility; she was the one who found the colon cancer in a place that others say would have gone undetected. She had a mission to complete and God allowed her to be there for me. God has a way of placing people in your life at the time you need them. After looking at the bigger picture, I realized that God had my back from the beginning. I explained to the assistant what was going on and she placed me on hold to speak with the doctor. When she returned she placed the doctor on the telephone and I began to re-explain what I had previously stated to the assistant. He asked me if I could come in after my treatment but before 1pm and I said yes. After my treatment I dashed nervously to the gastroenterologist. I began to pray and ask God to take away all fear and doubt. As I drove to the doctor I felt at peace. Those unexpected detours and obstacles in life can really play a number on you if you let it. And as stated in the previous chapters that during those times in your life learn to change your thought pattern (think positive) and lean on God.

When I reached the new doctor for consultation, he informed me that he did not see patients on Friday but had made an exception for me because he could hear the concern in my voice. He said he did not want me to spend the entire weekend worrying. Once again God was at work and He had my back. He had already had all of my the test results, blood work and mammogram results sent immediately to him and had reviewed them before I had arrived. He informed me that the normal CEA level is five and my level was at seven which was not too alarming. He stated that it could be a fluke with the blood test or that something could be going on in the colon but he doubted it very much. I had my colonoscopy that Monday and thank God the doctor informed me that from what he could see nothing was going on. He stated that he had removed two (2) flat polyps and he was sending them to the lab for a biopsy but he felt confident that all was well and would have to wait for the pathology report to confirm his findings. If you live long enough you will experience life and the unexpected obstacles which may occur. How you deal with it will determine your outcome. When you are running in a race you can't simply say I am going to run in a race, you have to train and prepare for it; if you don't prepare for it, it can be detrimental to you.

You have to prepare mentally and physically for the run. And such is life; you have to prepare yourself mentally and physically in different aspects of your life.

Let me give you an example, my sons wanted to play football so badly. Because they watched the game on television and played in the back yard they thought they could just join a team and play. When we signed them with a real team they began to see that there was more to it than just playing football. It was a routine; a rigorous routine I may add; they had to run laps, stretch, exercise and really learn how to play the game. Although they knew the plays and the calls they had to prepare to play the game by getting in shape.

4ask.healthline.com

The first year of playing football they picked up on the game but the teams were not winning many games.

They became discouraged at times and they wanted to give up. George and I began to talk to them and encourage them that giving up were not an option because they both had such a passion for the game. We told them that quitters never win and in spite what it looked like they were still winners. We told them that when things get tough you don't give up but push forward; push past their feelings. You have to instill confidence and self-esteem into children at an early age; teaching them not to give up and let them know that giving up is not an option. They may not understand it at the moment but they will understand it over time. The second year rolled around and they continued the rigorous routine and they continued to play the game; just as I stayed in the race with my treatments. My husband began to coach the team and then he begun to impart the same dialogue we had with our sons to the team. He began to express to the team the art of being positive and playing hard, showing up for practice and giving it your all. He along with another coach was able to bring this underdog team around. Would you believe, the team played hard and began to win every game? They became undefeated and guess what? They made it to the playoffs. Let me take it a step further they made it to the playoffs and won the championship game 40-0!! This was the underdog team who came out on top! Had they decided to give up they would have missed out on a great season, a great opportunity. All of their preparations paid off. You may ask why are you sharing this Sharon, are you gloating, no. I said all of that to say that when the tough gets going you don't give up or give in; you persevere. You persevere through the pain and through the aggravation like that of the saying "No pain, no gain!" Before you begin any race you have to prepare and I urge you to prepare yourselves mentally and physically for the obstacles that may occur in your life. You may ask the question, how do you prepare for these obstacles? Just as a runner prepares for the run by getting in shape and training, you prepare for life's obstacles by clearing your mind, praying and believing that whatever you are to face you will be alright. Don't you know that your thoughts affect your body; it has a trickling affect. Proverbs 23:7 speaks on this wise, what you think is what will be.

## Proverbs 23:7
### For as he thinketh in his heart, so is he:......

Whatever you are facing whether it be a bad report from the doctor, an unforeseen circumstance, etc. you have to prepare yourself mentally and physically for the challenge. Once you face the challenge, your race has thus begun. Be sure to gear your mind up with positive thoughts and pray constantly.

## Acts 6:4
### But we will give ourselves continually to prayer, and to the ministry of the word.

When you are officially in the race, you must continue; do not look at the distance or the obstacles ahead but concentrate on the outcome. You have to run to obtain what is waiting for you at the end, your healing; your victory; your win. Just like my sons in football if you hang in there and continue on you can become the champion of your situation. While running in the my race let me reiterate I totally wanted to give up at times but God who was the source of my strength gave me the courage to go on. You must go all the way to the end; don't give up. As stated in one of the previous chapters sometimes we give up too soon; if you hang in there a little while longer you will see that your victory is closer than you think.

We all have hurdles or crossroads in life; how you endure it will either make you or break you. Do not allow your spirit to be broken, do not allow negative thoughts or conversations to overtake your mind, do not allow the enemy to toy with you. You can and will break free of your circumstances if you allow God to be the source of your strength. Go forth in freedom, freedom from sickness, freedom from depression, freedom from drug addiction, freedom from whatever has you in bondage. Break free, with God's help you can be free and stay free!!! Once you are free stand firm in your freedom and do not allow yourselves to get caught in bondage again. Free your mind; change some things!

## John 8:36
### If the Son therefore shall make you free, ye shall be free indeed.

**The Importance of Believing**

While running in the race you must believe that you can complete the race. When you are facing life's challenges you have to believe the situation will turn out alright. In essence you must believe in something or someone. Upon doing research on believing *Tony Robbins put it so eloquently: Beliefs have the power to create and the power to destroy. Human beings have the awesome ability to take any experience of their lives and create a meaning that disempowers them or one that can literally saves their lives.*

How true that statement is. We have the power. God has given us that power.

I want to spend a little time stressing the importance of believing. 5Dictionary.com defines believing as (used without object, believed, believing -- To have confidence in truth, the existence, or the reliability of something, although without absolute proof that one is right in doing so. *"Only if one believes in something can one act purposefully."*
Verb phrases:
to have faith in the reliability, honesty, benevolence, etc., of :
*"I can help only if you believe in me."*
While reading the definition of believing on dictionary.com it gives an example of a very important factor, it reads and I quote: *"I can help only if you believe in me"*. That alone is a very powerful statement, let us re-read those words again slowly and carefully. ***"I can help only if you believe in me"***. In order to make something happen you have to first believe in something or someone. Believing in something or someone gives you that push and the zeal to go on or that desire to make it happen. At times depending upon the circumstances we are facing, we lose faith, lose hope and our ability to believe becomes clouded with our doubts, fears and concerns. The faith we once had is replaced by fear; fear of the unknown; fear of the what ifs. But when we believe in someone or something it gives you the extra push you need to continue. Some of you believe in a higher power, a higher being as some of you might call it. I believe in a higher power, a higher being and His name is Jesus (God). Believing coupled with God's spirit is the recipe for victory. God's spirit will uplift you when you are down and guide you in uncertainty. God is a lifter upper!!! Believing in God brings peace in your situation. Yes we

are human and we will be tested and our faith will be shaken but God will give you the peace that surpasses all understanding. I am a witness! Going back to the example, *"I can help only if you believe in me."* I want to rephrase this just a little, **God can help you if you believe in Him**, and it's just that simple. I am not trying to push my beliefs on you I just want you to look at the big picture. I thank God that I believe in Him, it was Him who has bought me to this point in my life. Without Him I could have lost my mind being diagnosed cancer twice in the same year. I will be honest it was not always easy during my ordeal, but I put my total trust in God and He saw me through.

Let me reiterate God can help you if you believe in Him.

### Philippians 4:7

**And the peace of God, which passeth all understanding, shall keep your hearts and minds through Christ Jesus.**

When you believe in God you gain added strength in your day to day life. God gives you the strength you need; in weakness you are made strong.

### II Corinthians 12:9

**And he said unto me, My grace is sufficient for thee: for my strength is made perfect in weakness.**

When you believe in God you have God's strength added to your own strength no matter how little of it you have; the two strengths together can be very powerful. You will be surprised that sometimes that added strength lifts you out of the slump you may be in. That strength can push us toward greatness, push us toward the victory and every so often that strength carries us to higher ground and or a higher place in God. God's strength gives us the power to accomplish miracles in our lives and in the lives of others. Let us walk this journey of life together knowing that God is with us, He can bring you out of your circumstance no matter how big or how small. Throughout this book I have spoken of God's goodness, I have encouraged you to move toward your victory. I wrote this for you and I wrote it for me.

After writing about how important it is to believe in something, it is as equally important to walk in what you believe in without wavering as stated in Hebrews 10:23 and James 1:6

## Hebrews 10:23
**Let us hold fast the profession of our faith without wavering; (for he is faithful that promised;)**

## James 1:6
**But let him ask in faith, nothing wavering. For he that wavereth is like a wave of the sea driven with the wind and tossed.**

While believing one must stand firm that victory is coming, no matter how it looks. I had to learn how to stand firmly on God and His Word and believe that victory was coming.

As I've mentioned previously, you really don't know how much strength you have until you are in an actual dilemma. I had to learn to push past the pain, push through the tears and keep on moving; keep on running. No matter how I felt I had to push, push, push. I pushed, I went to work, church, and my boys' games when I was able to; I had to take a stand!

As previously stated I went to work whenever my body allowed me to although at times I was extremely fatigued and experienced body aches but I pressed on anyway. My faith and my belief kept me pushing. One day as I was riding the train with a young lady, who I would see frequently, we began to converse about life and we shared our stories about what we were currently going through. She shared with me how she was battling leukemia and had to undergo bone marrows which were very painful and I shared with her that I was diagnosed with colon cancer in the beginning of 2013 and in the middle of 2013 diagnosed with breast cancer and undergoing chemotherapy. As we shared our stories she stated that she would have never imagined that I was diagnosed with cancer and or under-going chemotherapy treatments. She mentioned that my outer appearance would have never told the story of what I was currently experiencing and I always seemed to be in good spirits. After hearing my story she stated that she was uplifted and knew that she too was going to be alright. After we shared our stories that day I did not see her again for a while. Finally after some time we finally saw each other again. She began to tell me how she had just spoke about me the day before to a couple of her colleagues. She was saying that her colleagues always complained about everything. She went on to say that she took herself out of the equation because they knew about her situation and mentioned to them that she knew a young lady who was diagnosed with colon and breast cancer and in our conversations she never once heard me complain. She told them if the young lady could go through that and not complain how they could complain about the little simple things in life that are so minor. She asked them what they would do in a really bad situation. She said her colleagues agreed with what she was saying. Believing and walking in faith can uplift others. It is great when you can actually walk the talk and cause others to be uplifted and moved by your actions. Imagine if I was complaining to her about my situation and yet telling her that God is a healer, my actions would not line up with my walk. Instead my actions (my belief) and my walk were in line and she was able to share my story with someone else with hopes that they received the message to stop complaining and learn to move pass their circumstances. I am grateful to be the vessel that God used; as always I want God to get the glory out of my circumstance.

**Getting Closer to the Finish Line**

I am still in the race, two more treatments to go. I am running, running, running. As I look back the journey had been long but I was finally closer to the end. I was filled with excitement and anticipation.


**The Final Day**

By no means was it an ordinary day; it was the final day of treatment completion. I awoke looking forward to treatment. This was no ordinary day although George and I began our regular routine the same routine we dis day in and day out. As usual our days begin early, beginning with getting our sons, George and Chase ready for school. "It's time to get up", I said to the boys as I entered their rooms. "Get up, get up", they began to move slowly as they both rose to get up. As they began to assemble themselves for school, I walked downstairs to the kitchen to prepare breakfast and snacks. After the boys were dressed they hurried into the kitchen to have breakfast. "Your bus will be here soon so let's go", I uttered. Once the boys were done they waited for the school bus, within minutes the bus arrived and off went the boys to school. (Sounds familiar)

Instead of climbing back in bed I had to take time to pray and thank God for bringing me to this point. I certainly did not do it on my own and certainly no goodness of my own, it was God who gave me the strength to endure. I thank God for His goodness and mercy

## Psalms 23:6

**Surely goodness and mercy shall follow me all the days of my life: and I will dwell in the house of the LORD for ever.**

As I assembled myself for my very last chemotherapy treatment I was filled with emotions, I wanted to cry and laugh at the same time. God had brought me a mighty long way; one year and three months of chemotherapy treatments; thirty-eight sessions of radiation treatments and various tests in between. My end for chemotherapy treatments had finally come. I was overwhelmed. My oncologist as well as the staff at the center where I was administered the chemotherapy was exceptional; they were warm, compassionate and caring. I am grateful to God for placing them in my path for a season. There is a season for everything as mentioned in Ecclesiastes 3

## Ecclesiastes 3:1-8

**[1]To every thing there is a season, and a time to every purpose under the heaven:[2] A time to be born, and a time to die; a time to plant, and a time to pluck up that which is planted;[3] A time to kill, and a time to heal; a time to break down,**

and a time to build up;[4] A time to weep, and a time to laugh; a time to mourn, and a time to dance;[5] A time to cast away stones, and a time to gather stones together; a time to embrace, and a time to refrain from embracing;[6] A time to get, and a time to lose; a time to keep, and a time to cast away;[7] A time to rend, and a time to sew; a time to keep silence, and a time to speak;[8] A time to love, and a time to hate; a time of war, and a time of peace.

### I Had My Time

I had my time of weeping and God dried my tears away,
I had my time of sickness, and God healed me, I can say
this without dismay,
I had my time of breakdown and now it's my time to build
up again,
I had my time to pray,
While on other days I could not,
Thank God for stored up prayers.
I had my time of dark and weary days,
And I tried my best not to complain,
I knew at the end I would not go insane.
God had kept my mind,
Because it was Him who would bless me in His own time.
I had my time to keep silent
And now I have to speak,
And tell everyone I meet,
That Christ is real.
And yes He stills heals.

Written By Me For You

When I completed with my last chemotherapy treatment, I felt like I could conquer the world. The journey I traveled was finally over. I could now begin to concentrate on rebuilding myself and moving forward in this journey of life. I was elated that I was done and was declared **CANCER FREE**. Although I could not celebrate the way I wanted to after treatment because I was not feeling too well but knowing that it was my last treatment was celebration within itself. My God had proven Himself to me and for that I was grateful.

As I approach the next chapter of this book I pray that thus far you have been uplifted and blessed by my writings. I pray that a seed has been planted and embedded in your spirit that seed will manifest when you are faced with life's challenges. As I continue onto the next chapters I want to encourage you once again to not only endure as discussed in chapter 3, but to couple your endurance with believing the promises of God and totally putting your trust in Him.

# In Sickness and In Health

I Corinthians 7:3
Let the husband render unto the wife due
benevolence: and likewise also the wife unto the
husband.

# Chapter 4
## In Sickness and In Health
## Through A Husband's Eyes

Wedding vows are an integral part of the wedding ceremony. It is the part of the ceremony where two people vow to love each other no matter what. As I reminisce on our wedding vows: I George Robinson take one Sharon to be my wife, to have and to hold from this day forward, (Sept. 8, 1990), for better or for worse, for richer, for poorer, in **SICKNESS** and in health, to love and to cherish from this day forward (Sept. 8, 1990) until death us do part. We both responded to those vows by stating" I do". I took my vows very serious and meant every word. I promised to love my wife no matter what. Not knowing what the future had in store for us we could make it through anything as long as we love and treasure the commitment we made to each other. I vowed to love Sharon in sickness and in health and to be there for her. In sickness and in health are these just empty words of tradition or do they represent a lifetime commitment to the one you vowed them to? The longevity and quality of your marriage depends on it! I have seen on television and have heard numerous stories where men preferably husbands who when faced with adversity in their marriages run the other way. As I sat in the doctor's office and heard the doctor say, "You have been diagnosed with colon cancer" my heart skipped a beat. I could not believe what I was hearing; could this be a bad dream? Was I going to wake up from this terrible nightmare. As I sat there I realized that what the doctor was saying was real. I sat there in disbelief and thought to myself I don't want to lose my wife, we need to grow old together, raise our children together; we have to fight! I had to maintain my composure and be strong for Sharon. I looked at Sharon's face and although she seemed frightened by it all she was calm and attentive to what the doctor was saying.

Why couldn't this be me instead of her I thought to myself? I had so many mixed emotions going on in my head. I was not going to be that man who runs away from adversity. I was going to be there for my wife and fight for her healing. When I heard the diagnosis it was at that point in sickness and in health came alive. I had to man up and be there for her just as I was with her in good health. As we left the doctor's office I recall us walking to the car like zombies. I had to snap out of it and give my wife some words of encouragement. I remember telling her that all was going to be alright, God was not going to abandon us; He was going to see us through this. Once we digested the news we were able to talk about it more and figure out when would be the best time to tell close family and friends. I suggested that it would be best to meet with the surgeon first, get all of the necessary information and see what our options were going to be before we share the news. So that's what we did! In the meantime I remained prayerful because I knew from all my teachings, preaching and praying that God could do anything but fail and this situation was not too hard for God to handle. I hung on to what I believed in with all my might. After we received the information from the doctor and knew when the surgery was going to occur, we told our family and friends the news together. It was one of the hardest things I ever had to do. Sharon was calm during the entire ordeal. Her mental and spiritual state was incredible. In weakness you are surely made strong and strong she was.

The surgery went well and we were told that the cancer had not spread. Initially we thought Sharon would have to undergo chemotherapy and/or radiation but thank God she did not. She was well on her way to recovery and I thank God for bringing us out. We had made it through this test of life.

Approximately five months had passed and after a mammogram test we found ourselves in similar dilemma, Sharon now being diagnosed with breast cancer. Here it is I was experiencing it all over again, it felt like déjà vu, my God what's going on here I thought. Did the cancer spread I remember thinking to myself. I felt yet again that I was in a bad dream and waiting to be pinched so that I could awake. I must admit I was frightened because I didn't know what was really going on in her body. Once again I had to compose myself and be strong for my wife. I remember telling her that if God did it before, He can truly do it again. We had to be on one accord and believe that God was going to heal her once again. This time was different than the last, after the surgery and meeting with the oncologist we were told that Sharon had to undergo chemotherapy and radiation and that was news we did not want to hear. We had heard so many negative stories about the treatments and we were not happy about the news. Sickness and health became so surreal! My commitment to my wife came quickly into play once again. Charles Swindell put it so eloquently, commitment is a mindset, an attitude; a way of thinking that will enable you and your spouse to navigate through the test and storms of a marriage. He compared working on a marriage to remodeling a house:
- It takes longer than you plan
- It cost more than you figured
- It requires greater determination than you expected and sometimes the only thing that keeps us going is hope!

Hope is what kept us going. I thank God for hope. During this second ordeal it taught me patience to endure, experience in the circumstance and above all it gave us the hope we needed to make it through.

## Romans 5:4
## And patience, experience; and
## experience, hope:

What is hope? Dictionary.search.yahoo.com defines hope (Verb) as to have confidence; trust;
Noun: The longing or desire for something accompanied by the belief in the possibility of its occurrence. Hope accompanied with faith got us through. Although we did not see with our human eyes the victory but with our spiritual eye we saw victory ahead.

## Hebrews 11:1
## Now faith is the substance of things hoped for, the evidence of things not seen.

It is hard as a man to see anyone suffering or going through pain but when it's your wife it's so different. My wife is the backbone of our marriage and I could not believe what was happening. Words cannot really describe how my heart was aching. I did not want to see my wife go through the pain of chemotherapy or radiation. I had to brace myself for what was coming ahead. I prayed and asked God to be with Sharon and take her through her treatments. I asked God to be our strength and importantly heal her yet again. I had to cling to my belief and my faith. I can remember the first day of treatment so well, we went to treatment not knowing what to expect but we anticipated that God was going to take her through. As we walked into the building I prayed like never before. Once we met with the oncologist and Sharon was cleared for chemotherapy I still did not know what to expect; this was her first time experiencing chemotherapy and we were nervous. When the nurse first administered the chemotherapy intravenously; I thought to myself wow so this is how chemo works! Sharon was a trooper and was so calm during the whole ordeal. She asked questions and listened tentatively to the administering nurse. After a few treatments, she began to get sick, she was extremely fatigue, had loss of appetite and weight loss. After a few treatments Sharon lost all of her hair although devastated at first she embraced it and acted as if nothing had happened. As I watched all of this unfold before my eyes, I thought to myself, my wife is amazing. My amazing wife although she was not feeling her best still tried to maintain the house and do her wifely duties. She did not let it get her too down. Don't get me wrong she had some bad days; I encouraged her, held her and upheld her in prayer. Because of my commitment to her and our family, I picked up the slack of when necessary and was proud to do so. It is such a blessing when you are able to be there for your family. Chemotherapy and radiation treatments were long and hard but with God on our side, we got through it together. It was as if I felt my wife's pain; you see when she hurts I hurt too. We have a bond that could never be broken.

I want to take this opportunity to say to every man reading this book or this chapter, encourage your wife not only in good times but in bad times. We are all faced with adversity at some point in our lives and we must man up and take responsibility.

### A Husband's Role

- As a husband you must take your role as the leader of your household. It is as clear cut as I can get, stand up and take your rightful positon. You are the head of your household so lead. When you lead be sure to lead by example; if you have children they are watching what you do.

## Ephesians 5:23
## For the husband is the head of the wife, even as Christ is the head of the church: and he is the saviour of the body.

- Love your wife unconditionally and by that I mean love her without condition, love her as she is with no limitations. You had to see something in her that is why you married her in the first place. Love her regardless if you cannot see the higher picture of divine order. God has your back if you learn to pray and take Him at His word.

## Ephesians 5:25
## Husbands, love your wives, even as Christ also loved the church, and gave himself for it;

- Let her know verbally that you value her, adore her, respect her and love her. As men we go about our day and oftentimes we become so relaxed in our skins that we do not verbally tell our wives that we love them because we feel they already know it. But we must keep that communication line open and express our love to them. I am guilty of this and I am working on it too.

- Serve your wife, I know some of you are saying what are you talking about George, you have gone too far now!!! You are still the head of your house; being the head of your house does not necessarily mean being her master, but her servant. One of the best ways to serve your wife is to understand her and her needs and try to meet those needs. Be that listening ear if she needs to vent. We have young children yes we were late bloomers but I know she needs assistance with our boys' homework, housework at times or whatever needs she may have. I try to assist whenever and wherever I can. We are a team. When she was undergoing her treatments I had to pick up the slack to assist and I did not mind at all. Another way to serve your wife is to provide for her, this is one of the responsibilities and by this I mean assuming responsibility for meeting the material needs of your family. The word of God is a great road map; it will lead you and help you navigate through the cares of life. I Timothy 5:8 tells us that if anyone does not provide for his own especially those in his household is worse than an unbeliever. Just as you provide for her material needs of the family you must provide and take the initiative in helping her meet her spiritual needs as well. You do this by modeling Godly character, by praying with her and for her, spending time together in God's Word and looking for ways to encourage her spiritually.

## 1 Timothy 5:8
**But if any provide not for his own, and specially for those of his own house, he hath denied the faith, and is worse than an infidel.**

Let me ask a question, do you know what your wife's top two or three needs are right now?  Right now what is she worried about?  What seems to be troubling her and what pressure is she currently under?  As her husband, learn the answers to particular questions like this and then do what you can to reduce her worries, her troubles, and her pressures.  Run her bath every now and then, make her feel like the queen she is.  As a matter of fact she is the queen of your household and yes you are the king!

- Lastly be a Lover not a Fighter, I read a poster the other day and it read:  Be a Lover Not a Fighter But Always Fight For What You Love.  Oh how true that statement is; how many times have we fought for things we wanted whether it is trying to gather money for that new car or trying to get that promotion on your job.  If you can fight for those kinds of things why not fight for the woman you love.  Loving is much easier than fighting and it can be fun too.  You will have disagreements but learn from those disagreements and move forward.  Do not dwell on the past but concentrate and move toward the future.  Your future is brighter and better.  Better days are coming, I promise!

To be a true leader of your household, lover, and a servant is to submit your life to the gift God has given you—your wife.  My wife and I will be celebrating our 25th wedding anniversary in September 2015, although at times our lives were thrown curve balls we knew when to duck and when to pray.  We had our ups and downs as any married couple would but we learned how to persevere.  As previously mentioned when she was diagnosed with cancer we knew what we had to do.  We had to come together as a unit and pray that God would bless and heal her and God came through for us.  Watching her go through her medical ordeal has given us the strength we never knew we had. Together with God and prayer we can move mountains. You too can have the power to move mountains with your spouse if you allow God to take charge over your circumstance. I am a witness. I say to you if your wife has been diagnosed with a condition remember she does not have to die with it, the Word of God says I will live and not die.

## Psalm 118:17
### I shall not die, but live, and declare the works of the LORD.

She will live and she too can be a Survivor. My wife asked a question in the beginning of this book, is there anything too hard for God and my answer to you is no. God can give peace in chaos and give you a solution to your problem. Allow God to be God over your life.

# Believing the Promise

Galatians 3:14
That the blessing of Abraham might come on the
Gentiles through Jesus Christ; that we might
receive the **promise of** the Spirit through faith.

.

# Chapter 5
## Believing the Promise

What is a **promise**? A promise is defined in the Webster's II New College Dictionary as follows: An assurance that one will or will not do something; to provide a basis for expecting.

When a person makes a promise he is giving his word that he will fulfill it or not fulfill it. People make promises everyday and people sometimes break promises. Below are some examples of promises that different people might make:

A) "Can I borrow $10.00 I promise I'll pay you back tomorrow."

B) "Mom and Dad, I will do better on my next report card, I promise"

C) "I ll be sure to pray for you."

D) "Mom I promise I will clean my room in a minute"

E) "I promise I will be there in 10 minutes"

Some of you have probably made some of these same promises and broken a few of them too. Many times people break their promises and they must take full responsibility for it. Maybe they forgot, maybe they changed their mind or maybe they just failed to do what they said they would do. Sometimes people break their promises because of circumstances and situations beyond their control (bad weather, a flat tire, sickness, etc.). Are there any circumstances that are beyond God's control? Does God say, "I wanted to keep that promise but something unexpected came up and I was not able to"? And the answer is No; God will fulfill His promise. Many of God's promises are conditional which means that God promises to do something **IF** man does something. For example a parent might give a conditional promise to their child: "**IF**" you finish all of the vegetables on your plate, you can have dessert!" You see the child had to do something to receive the promise; the dessert. "**IF**" we do our part, God will do His part. "**IF**" we believe that God can perform His promise, we can have whatsoever we ask. We must be persuaded in our minds that God can do it.

### Romans 8:21
### And being fully persuaded that, what he had promised, he was able to perform.

God also has unconditional promises, which mean when God gives an unconditional promise, there are no "if's," "and's," or "but's" about it, God says, "I WILL DO SOMETHING" and it does not matter if man likes it or not, believe it or not--God is still going to do it! GOD WILL do what He promised no matter what, that is an unconditional promise. An unconditional promise has no stipulations or conditions. An example of the unconditional promise is found in Genesis 9:8-11. In this text God makes an unconditional promise that He will never again destroy the earth with a flood again like found in Genesis 6:8. Unconditional promises are simply God's declaration of His commitment to act in a certain way. There are many such promises in the Bible. There are some things that God is just going to do. God will fulfill his promises He cannot lie.

### Hebrews 6:18
### That by two immutable things, in which it was impossible for God to lie, we might have a strong consolation, who have fled for refuge to lay hold upon the hope set before us.

God's conditional and unconditional promises do us no good unless we believe them. In Hebrews 4:1-2, the children of Israel were given a promise but they did not believe the promise. God's Word will not profit us unless we continue to read the next verse of Hebrews 4:1, verse 2. You must mix God's Word and your faith in order to achieve victory. Again if you do something God will do something,

## Hebrews 4:1-2
**₁Let us therefore fear, lest, a promise being left us of entering into his rest, any of you should seem to come short of it.**
**₂For unto us was the gospel preached as well as unto them: but the word preached did not profit them, not being mixed with faith in them that heard it.**

Think of food when you are hungry; your refrigerator is full of all the foods you want to eat but it has to be cooked first. It profits you nothing if you do not cook the food using all the necessary ingredients and nutrients to satisfy your hunger. God's Word is like that, it is there to minister to us and feed our spiritual man and increase our faith in God. We must take God at His Word in order for our faith to be increased. It profits us nothing unless we use the Word and apply the Word to our daily lives.

## II Corinthians 9:10
**Now he that ministereth seed to the sower both minister bread for your food, and multiply your**

**seed sown, and increase the fruits of your righteousness;**

I have learned that God's promises are sure. His Word has come out of His mouth and will not return to you void. During my medical ordeals God had proved Himself to me and fulfilled His promise to me that I shall live and not die. And I shall live to tell you of those promises.

## Isaiah 55:11
**So shall my word be that goeth forth out of my mouth: it shall not return unto me void, but it accomplish that which I please, and it shall prosper in the thing whereto I sent it.**

## Psalms 118:17
**I shall not die, but live, and declare the works of the LORD.**

Experiencing trauma, sickness or any curveball that life throws at us doesn't simply condemn us to a life of suffering and helplessness. Instead, we can pull strength, courage, and wisdom out of misfortune after having been caught in it. If I had not gone through my experiences, I would not be where I am today. I would not have written this book to encourage you and to let you know that you have the strength to endure your experiences. I would not be able to tell you while in your race of life not to focus on the finish line but continue to run with patience so that you can receive all the blessings along the path. While running the race, you will pick up so many blessings: strength, endurance, humility and appreciation. You are champions in my eyes but especially in the eyes of God. Go forth and be that Goliath. Everyone is familiar with the story of David and Goliath and how David, the underdog became the true champion. Regardless of your circumstances you have to fight like Goliath and push forward and while pushing forward you must believe that you will be alright. You can read I Samuel 17 on David and Goliath. Don't you know that great odds can be overcome by underdogs especially if the motivation is strong enough? With God on your side, you will win even if the odds are against you. I have learned that experiencing adversity not only equips you to deal with negative events but helps us appreciate the positive ones, possibly increasing our overall satisfaction with life. Sometimes we take little things for granted and when you are faced with adversity you have a greater appreciation for life.

## 1 Samuel 17:4
## And there went out a champion out of the camp of the Philistines, named Goliath, of Gath, whose height was six cubits and a span.

When I was undergoing chemotherapy treatment I tried not to concentrate on how I felt. I tried to remain as positive and prayerful as possible in order to gain that inner peace I needed to make it another day. Whatever you are facing I once again encourage you to be positive and think positive. I recall a sermon by my pastor entitled "A Positive Person Will Always Conquer", where he basically spoke about how a positive thinking person will always succeed; the key to it all is being positive and taking God at His Word. The bible is our road map and it's up to us to decide which road we would travel; will it be the positive road or the negative road. The choice is yours.

Whatever situation you are previously facing as previously chapters you must first change your thought pattern. You have to be positive and not allow the enemy to flood your mind with negativity. Proverbs 23:7 states for as a man thinketh in his heart so he is. If you think negative thoughts, negativity will consume you. In math, a negative plus a negative equals a negative ( - + - = - ); a negative cannot produce a positive on its own. In some instances like in math when a person receives the negative report from the doctor, they allow the negative thoughts to overtake them. They concentrate on the illness instead of concentrating on getting better.

In some instances the negativity of the illness kills a person and not the actual sickness. Sometimes we give up too soon; it seems easier to give up than to fight. We must think positive and have faith in God for our healing. The two go hand and hand. Positive Thinking + Faith in God = Blessings.

## Proverbs 23:7
## For as he thinketh in his heart, so is he......

I wrote about the promises of God and believing those promises can be difficult especially when you are in the actual struggle. But while in the struggle not only does one have to believe you must have faith that all is going to be well. We must learn to be like Abraham. God bestowed on Abraham all the promises He promised to give because he had faith and confidence in Him. Faith became an integral part of Abraham's character. He had a heart for God and obeyed Him. Faith automatically builds a strong relationship and fellowship with God. We, too, should have faith in God because through faith we are justified and receive the promises God made to Abraham.  Don't you know we are heirs of Abraham!

## Genesis 26:4-5
**4And I will make thy seed to multiply as the stars of heaven, and will give unto thy seed all these countries; and in thy seed shall all the nations of the earth be blessed.  5Because that Abraham obeyed my voice, and kept my charge, my commandments, my statues, and my laws.**

## Galatians 3:16
**Now to Abraham and his seed were the promises made…..**

If we can have the faith the size of a mustard seed and believe that God will fulfill His promises, He promised to us then we are on our way to being like Abraham.  We need to exercise the same faith that Abraham exercised.   God's promise is promised to us, our children, our children's children and so on and so forth.   I had to believe the promise that God was going to completely heal not only me but my son.  "I will be cancer free, cancer will not return anywhere in my body; my son will be healed of Bell's palsy and we both will never have these conditions again in Jesus' name.  What God has promised He will and is able to accomplish.  I thank God that I can now testify that if you believe on the promises of God He can heal, He can set free, He can deliver.

## Matthew 17:20
**He replied, "Because you have so little faith.**

Truly I tell you, if you have faith as small as a mustard seed, you can say to this mountain, 'Move from here to there,' and it will move. Nothing will be impossible for you."

**Acts 2:39**

**For the promise is unto you, and to your children, and to all that are afar off, even as many as the Lord our God shall call.**

Let me speak briefly about the promise God made to Abraham; Abraham's wife Sarai was barren and had past her age to conceive. What does barren mean? [1]Yahoo dictionary's meaning of barren is not producing or incapable of producing offspring. Used of women. In other words Sarai was not capable of having children. God spoke to Abraham giving him the most remarkable promise. The Lord said to Abram, "Go forth from your country, and from your relatives and from your father's house, to the land which I will show you; and I will make you a great nation, and I will bless you, and make your name great; and so you shall be a blessing; and I will bless those who bless you, and the one who curses you I will curse. And in you all the families of the earth shall be blessed" **(Genesis 12:1-3).** He promised Abraham a son through Sarai who was barren and his name was to be called Isaac. Not only did God promise Abraham a son but he renamed Abram to "Abraham" meaning "father of many", and gives Sarai a new name, "Sarah". Most of us want God to bless us NOW, but sometimes God allows us to go through the struggle to teach us how to wait; teach us who He really is and to strengthen our faith in Him. God may not come when we want Him to but He is always on time. Like Sara she was barren, but God blessed her to conceive even in her old age. We must learn to WAIT.

**Hebrews 11:11**
**Through faith also Sara herself received strength to conceive seed, and was delivered of a child when she was past age, because she judged him faithful who had promised.**

## *We Must Believe the Promises of God. Remember we are Heirs of Abraham!!*

### A Promise Delayed But Not Denied

I have previously written about a promise God made to Abraham and Sarai in Hebrews 11, Sara had two strikes against her 1) she was barren and 2) she was past her age to conceive. Although she had the odds against her, God kept His promise and blessed her to conceive. Another example of what God has done in my life. Back in the late 1990's I was diagnosed with endometriosis and was told by a doctor that I would not be able to conceive.

### [2]What is Endometriosis

When you have endometriosis, the type of tissue that lines your uterus is also growing outside your uterus. The clumps of tissue (called implants) may have grown on your ovaries or fallopian tubes, the outer wall of the uterus, the intestines, or other organs in the belly. In rare cases they spread to areas beyond the belly. Some women have no symptoms or problems. Others have mild to severe symptoms or infertility. There is no way to predict whether endometriosis will get worse, will improve, or will stay the same until menopause.

[1]Yahoodictionary.com
[2]Reference: WebMD.com

My husband and I began to fast and pray and believe that God was going to bless my womb. One Sunday morning I remember the sermon so well by Bishop James I. Clark; he took his text from Luke 1 and as he read the words from the bible, one verse came alive in my spirit, **Luke 1:37 For with God nothing shall be impossible.**

## Luke 1:37
## For with God nothing shall be impossible.

Bishop Clark's sermon was about Elizabeth who was barren and how God blessed her to conceive a son. As I sat in my seat and listened to him preach, he said these words, "there is nothing too hard for God". Those words resonated in my spirit. As he spoke I was compelled to read Luke 1 in its entirety every day and embed it into my spirit. As I read the scripture everyday something began to happen; within months I became pregnant. Although I had a miscarriage, God had done the impossible; he enabled me to conceive when the doctor said I would not be able to. It was a bittersweet test although at the time I did not know that God was preparing me for my blessing; the blessing of my two (2) sons.

## Luke 1:7, 13
**⁷ And they had no child, because that Elisabeth was barren, and they both were now well stricken in years.**
**¹³ But the angel said unto him, Fear not, Zacharias: for thy prayer is heard; and thy wife Elisabeth shall bear thee a son, and thou shalt call his name John.**

After having five miscarriages, one of which were twins, in 2002 and 2004, God honored my request, His promise and blessed me to have two healthy sons, George Cameron in 2002 and Chase Jarrett in 2004. I feel that I have to share the entire story with you because if God can bless me He can certainly bless you too. Someone is reading this and needs to hear this. So let me begin, I was approximately four months pregnant and began to experience some discomfort, cramping and bleeding. I was rushed to the hospital and while there I passed a large clot. Upon taking a Sonogram the technician saw no signs of a heartbeat or my son. He said I probably had a miscarriage and needed to schedule an appointment with my OB/GYN doctor for further instructions. I remember telling my husband that I thought it was in our best interest not to try again to have any children and that perhaps we should adopt or it will remain the two of us. It had become too painful for the both of us, the back and forth to the hospital and the miscarriages. Some tine had passed, it was around the Christmas holidays and I continued my regular routine. My mind was completely made up that we were not going to have any children and I was fine with that. It took some time to get in that frame of mind but I had to in order to go on. So my husband and I discussed the possibility of adoption and we spoke with a woman in our church that worked with an adoption agency and she gave us some paper work to fill out as well as workshops that we had to attend.

After a few days I went to my medical doctor for a routine check-up and he explained to me that I needed to see my obstetrician for a possible Dilation and Curettage (D&C) procedure because my HCG blood levels were very high and that I possibly needed a scrapping.

### 3What is a Dilation and Curettage

A Dilation and Curettage (D&C) is a brief surgical procedure in which the cervix is dilated and a special instrument is used to scrape the uterine lining. Knowing what to expect before, during, and after a D&C may help ease your worries and make the process go more smoothly. Here's what you need to know.

### 4You may need a D&C for one of several reasons. It's done to:

- Remove tissue in the uterus during or after a miscarriage or abortion or to remove small pieces of placenta after childbirth. This helps prevent infection or heavy bleeding.
- Diagnose or treat abnormal uterine bleeding. A D&C may help diagnose or treat growths such as fibroids, polyps, or endometriosis, hormonal imbalances, or uterine cancer. A sample of uterine tissue is viewed under a microscope to check for abnormal cells.

### What is HCG?

HCG is the abbreviation for "Human Chorionic Gonadotropin," also known as the pregnancy hormone. This hormone is produced by the placenta as soon as implantation happens, about one week after fertilization and ovulation. HCG levels continue to rise after implantation until about 10-12 weeks gestation, at which point the HCG level will stabilize or drop.

I informed my doctor that I was unhappy with my current obstetrician because neither he nor the previous OB/GYN doctors could explain to me and my husband why I continued to have miscarriages. I explained to him that the problem was not that I couldn't conceive as he could see, the problem was carrying full-term. He referred me to a colleague of his who was an obstetrician, Dr. Monique Defour-Jones. He told me to call her immediately to schedule a possible Dilation and Curettage (D&C).

As soon as I returned home I called Dr. Jones immediately and she spoke directly to me. My medical doctor had spoken with her and given her the details of my situation. As I was explaining to her about my HGC levels being very high and actually giving her the exact numbers, she said something that amazed me, "You are still pregnant". I was in total disbelief and insisted that I was not still pregnant according to the sonogram I had received at the hospital. She asked me the name of the hospital and look at God she was affiliated with the Hospital. She told me that she was going to give the hospital a call to retrieve the report and she would get back to me as soon as she received the information. When God makes a promise He fulfills that promise. He never goes back on His Word. Within an hour I received a call from the doctor who requested that I see her right away so she could examine me. My husband and I rushed to her office not knowing what to expect but not getting our hopes up high and went with the expectation that I was not still pregnant.

3Reference: WebMD.com
4www.babymed.com

I began to discuss with her my previous miscarriage history. She said she wanted to get to the bottom line as to why I was not able to carry full term. Once we were done discussing my previous history; she then examined me and did a sonogram. Well to me and my husband's surprise as she did the sonogram there was a heartbeat, she turned up the volume so that we both can hear it loud and clear. I almost fell off the bed when I heard the heart beat! Not only did we hear the heart beat but we saw my son on the screen. What an experience to be first told that you had miscarried and a few weeks later to find out you're still pregnant. My husband and I were so excited. Sometimes we cannot explain the mysteries of God. He at times does things you least expect. He always seems to manifest Himself in awkward situations so that we are awed! And I was awwwed!!!!

## 1 Timothy 3:16
**And without controversy great is the mystery of godliness: God was manifest in the flesh, justified in the spirit, seen of angels, preached unto the gentiles, believed on in the world, received up into glory.**

Shortly after finding out that I was still pregnant we received a letter from the adoption agency inviting George and I to an Adoption Orientation meeting. Because I was under strict doctor's care we could not follow suit with the adoption plans and furthermore I was pregnant hoping to have a child of my own.

Dr. Jones had stated that she was going to get to the bottom of why I had miscarried in the past and during the course of my pregnancy I was diagnosed with an incompetent cervix which was causing me to have miscarriages. Once the baby would get to a certain weight my cervix could not carry the baby. Dr. Jones had gotten to the root of the problem. She was heaven sent. She told me that I needed to receive a cervix cerclage which will help me carry my baby. I received a cervix cerlage for both of my sons.

### 5What is an Incompetent Cervix

During pregnancy, as the baby grows and gets heavier, it presses on the cervix. This pressure may cause the cervix to start to open before the baby is ready to be born. This condition is called incompetent cervix or weakened cervix, and it may lead to a miscarriage or premature delivery. However, an incompetent cervix happens in only about 1 out of 100 pregnancies.

### What is a Cervical Cerclage

Cervical cerclage is the placement of stitches in the cervix to hold it closed. In select cases, this procedure is used to keep a weak cervix (incompetent cervix) from opening early. When a cervix opens early, it may cause pre-term labor and delivery. If you have an incompetent cervix, your doctor may recommend cervical cerclage.

5Reference: WebMD.com

Cervical cerclage involves stitching shut the cervix, which is the outlet of the uterus. Cerclage can be done preventively at 12 to 14 weeks before the cervix thins out, or as an emergency measure after the cervix has thinned. It is rarely used after 24 weeks.

Cerclage is performed using either general anesthesia or regional anesthesia (such as spinal injection). The surgery can be done in different ways:

- Stitches can be placed around the outside of the cervix.
- A special tape can be tied around the cervix and stitched in place.

- A small incision can be made in the cervix. A special tape is then tied through the cervix to close it.

A few weeks after the cerclage procedure, I began to have some complications and was hospitalized. I was in the hospital for 3 ½ months on extensive bed rest and had to lay partially upside down my entire stay. I was under strict orders from Dr. Jones and was not allowed to get out of bed to walk around or even use the rest room for the entire time I was hospitalized. It was not easy but I made good of the situation. I gained a good rapport with the doctors and nurses and was given a private room. My husband bought my computer and printer to my room and I was able to do work from my hospital bed. I continued to do God's work from my hospital bed too; I was able to plan a service and an event for the auxiliary I worked with. I even managed to do a couple of programs for some weddings that were coming up at the time. Dr. Jones was amazed at what I was accomplishing while lying in a hospital bed. I was determined to get my son here with the help of God and did what I had to do. With my second son I was hospitalized for two weeks and placed on bed rest at home for the duration of the pregnancy. God gave me the strength to endure not once but twice; it was not easy but I did it.

I am writing this testimony to encourage a woman reading this portion of this book, yes you; you turned specifically to this chapter so that I can encourage you and let you know that there is nothing too hard for God.

**Jeremiah 32:17**
**Ah Lord GOD! behold, thou hast made the**
**heaven and the earth by thy great power and**

## stretched out arm, and there is nothing too hard for thee:

You have tried over and over again to conceive and still nothing. Remember I was told by a doctor that I would never conceive but my husband and I continued to try. We tried for ten years and nothing happened for us. I was ready to throw in the towel, I went as far as getting adoption papers but even still God had my back. He did not allow me to throw in the towel. When the Word of God hit me that Sunday morning the word was embedded in my spirit: **For with God nothing shall be impossible. (Luke 1:37).** It was then I began to take God at His Word. I read that scripture continuously every day until something happened. God was doing the work in me and preparing me for my blessing. Although I had several miscarriages, at least at that point I knew I could conceive; now God had to complete the work he had begun.

6Reference: WebMD.com

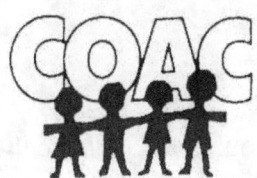

January 4, 2002

Ms. Sharon Robinson
████████████████

Dear Ms. Robinson:

Thank you for your recent inquiry about adopting through COAC. Your are invited to our next Adoption Orientation Meeting, which will be held on Wednesday, January 9, 2002 from 6:00 to 8:00 PM at 589 Eighth Avenue, 15th Floor.

We will look forward to seeing you at the meeting, which will be interesting and informative.

If you have any questions, please feel free to contact me at ████████████████

Yours very truly,

████████████████

Family Coordinator

I am speaking to you, *"you will receive the blessings that God has for you"*, but first you must say it and most importantly believe it. Don't look at the problem, look to the problem solver. God is capable of handling anything. The longer you wait the bigger your blessing! Hang in there!

## Deuteronomy 28:2
**And all these blessings shall come on thee, and overtake thee, if thou shalt hearken unto the voice of the LORD thy God.**

To build anything in life and/or to succeed at anything you must have an opposing force. Trials and tribulations are placed in our lives for a reason; although some trials and tribulations we create ourselves. We must have that opposing force to help make us strong and to build character. When a person wants to lose weight or build muscle, they exercise; some go to the gym while others do exercise at home to help them accomplish their goal. Exercising builds muscles, cardio, strength, and muscle tone, toning of the body, as well as wellness and health. The opposing force that most people encounter while trying to accomplish their goal is food, food and more food and not wanting on some days to exercise at all. But you must push forward to ensure that the goals you set for yourself are accomplished. Just like in the natural realm you have that opposing force, you experience it in the spiritual realm, the Word declares in

## Ephesians 6:12
**For we wrestle not against flesh and blood, but against principalities, against powers, against**

**the rulers of the darkness of this world, against spiritual wickedness in high places.**

Although we wrestle, in the end, we **WIN**!! Don't you know wrestling builds spiritual muscles where we are able to knock the devil out!! You can knock him out with:

1) The Word of God
2) Your Faith
3) The Strength to Endure the Test
4) The Courage To Go On

God has equipped you therefore use the tools God has given you. You are well equipped for the fight. Remember you must be fully covered. If you are covered the opposing force will not overtake you, you will overtake it. Don't forget, you're equipped!!

## Ephesians 6:11-18
**11Put on the whole armour of God, that ye may be able to stand against the wiles of the devil.**
**<sup>12</sup> For we wrestle not against flesh and blood, but against principalities, against powers, against the rulers of the darkness of this world, against spiritual wickedness in high places.**
**<sup>13</sup> Wherefore take unto you the whole armour of God, that ye may be able to withstand in the evil day, and having done all, to stand.**
**<sup>14</sup>Stand therefore, having your loins girt about with truth, and having on the breastplate of righteousness;**
**<sup>15</sup> And your feet shod with the preparation of the gospel of peace;**

**16 Above all, taking the shield of faith, wherewith ye shall be able to quench all the fiery darts of the wicked.**
**17 And take the helmet of salvation, and the sword of the Spirit, which is the word of God:**
**18 Praying always with all prayer and supplication in the Spirit, and watching thereunto with all perseverance and supplication for all saints;**

**1 Thessalonians 5:8**
**But let us, who are of the day, be sober, putting on the breastplate of faith and love; and for an helmet, the hope of salvation.**

The unexpected detours of life yes they came for me and yes they are coming for you if they have not come already, but I want you to be encouraged you are greater than your storm. My first real test of life came in 2000 when I had to fight for my son to be here and fight I did. God equipped me and I fought back. My second and third fight was in 2013-2014 my battle with cancer; I had to fight my life to live. While in this test I really got a chance to see the full manifestation of God in my life. I had to get to a level where I truly believed God, trusted Him and had faith in what He could do. I had to in order to endure and move forward. Although the struggles were not easy I gained strength I never knew I had. I want you to know that God is real, His power is real, healing is real, His Word is real. So count it all joy when you are going through your trial, for the trying of your faith worketh patience.

## James 1:2-4

2 **My brethren, count it all joy when ye fall into divers temptations; 3Knowing this that the trying of your faith worketh patience. 4But let patience have her perfect work, that ye may be perfect and entire, wanting nothing.**

In chapter 3 I spoke about approaching the finish line. While running closer to the finish line I could hear the cheers of the saints, family and friends, I could hear them say "Come on Sharon you can make it, look you are almost there". I could feel the energy of prayers that went forth for me and my family so I ran faster. I could feel the power of God and see the manifestation of God's Word and thus I ran harder. I may have lost some footage during the race, but I got back on track and kept running. I got tired, I even got weak but I kept running. I wanted to throw in the towel but I kept running. At some point I was able to see the finish line and was able to persevere. With God **I can do all things through Christ which strengtheneth me**. **(Philippians 4:13)** I was gaining ground so I had to endure to the end so I continued. You have to know that Victory was coming!!!

## Hebrews 12:1

**Wherefore seeing we also are compassed about with so great a cloud of witnesses, let us lay aside every weight, and the sin which doth so easily beset us, and let us run with patience the race that is set before us,**

**II Corinthians 12:9**

**And he said unto me, My grace is sufficient for thee: for my strength is made perfect in weakness. Most gladly therefore will I rather glory in my infirmities, that the power of Christ may rest upon me.**

Hold your ground, you are almost at your finish line too!

# Trust

Proverbs 3:5-6

**Trust** in the Lord with all thine heart; and lean not unto thine own understanding. In all thy ways acknowledge him, and he shall direct thy paths.

# Chapter 6
## The Power to Trust

After reading my book countless times before sending it to be published, I discussed in previous chapters faith, strength, the courage to endure and believing the promises of God in detail. And in order to obtain all of these "Trust" links all of this together.

In order to have faith, one must have TRUST,

In order to have strength and maintain strength, one must have TRUST,

In order to have courage, one must have TRUST and

In order to believe on the promises of God, one must have TRUST.

The key factor in all chapters is "TRUST".

Definition.com defines trust as a reliance on the integrity, strength, ability, surety, etc. of a person or thing, confidence. The Merriam Webster dictionary defines trust as belief that someone or something is reliable, good, honest, effective, etc.

Synonyms: certainty, belief, faith

**How Can We Trust**

We are able to trust someone based upon his or her character; a person's track record also plays an important role. A person's track record is based upon their integrity, honesty, faithfulness, and their ability to perform. We look at these aspects and it is then we make the determination that we can trust that individual. When I had my lumpectomy I trusted that the doctor would remove the cancerous tumor because he was the one who had the capabilities and the ability to perform this kind of surgery. He had done several lumpectomies before and his integrity spoke for itself therefore I felt confident enough to place my life in his hands. I trusted that God was going to bless the hands of the doctor and that He was going to bring me out.

## Who Can We Trust
We can search the pages of the scriptures and read countless times of those who trusted God. Men and women like Noah, Abraham, Moses, Job, Hannah, Elizabeth, and the list can go on and on. Trust once again is the surety of believing in someone or something who has the ability to perform. I know someone who fits this description, His name is Jesus, some call Him El Shaddai – The Lord Almighty, Some call Him Jehovah Rapha – The Lord That Heals, Some Call Him Jehovah Tsidkenu – The Lord Our Righteousness, Some Call Him Elohim – The Everlasting God, Some Call Him Jehova Jireh – The Lord will Provide. I simply call Him God. You can totally put your trust in Him because:
1. God is Reliable,
2. God is Able to Perform,
3. God is Good,
4. God is Faithful

## God's Good Track Record
God has a track record like no other. You can read about Jonah in the whale, Elizabeth who was barren, Job who lost everything and Mary and Martha who will influence you to put your trust in the one who rose again from the grave.
God's integrity speaks for itself, if He can raise Lazarus from the dead, what do you think He can do for you.
"Integrity is keeping a commitment even after circumstances have changed." ~ David Jeremiah

In the circumstance of Lazarus, he was dead, the dynamics had changed. God stayed where He was for two (2) days and did not rush to where Lazarus was laid because He had a point to make.  He is the almighty one and His timing is always on time.

### John 11:1-7, 21-22, 39-40, 43-44

1Now a certain man was sick, named Lazarus, of Bethany, the town of Mary and her sister Martha. 2(It was that Mary which anointed the Lord with ointment, and wiped his feet with her hair, whose brother Lazarus was sick.) 3Therefore his sisters sent unto him, saying, Lord, behold, he whom thou lovest is sick. 4When Jesus heard that, he said, This sickness is not unto death, but for the glory of God, that the Son of God might be glorified thereby. 5Now Jesus loved Martha, and her sister, and Lazarus. 6When he had heard therefore that he was sick, he abode two days still in the same place where he was. 7Then after that saith he to his disciples, Let us go into Judaea again.

21Then said Martha unto Jesus, Lord, if thou hadst been here, my brother had not died. 22 But I know, that even now, whatsoever thou wilt ask of God, God will give it.

39 Jesus said, Take ye away the stone. Martha, the sister of him that was dead, saith unto him, Lord, by this time he stinketh: for he hath been dead four days. 40 Jesus saith unto her, Said I

- Purifying your Mind - Renewing your thoughts; staying positive (Philippians 4:8)

**REMEMBER:** The Vibrations of your thoughts can affect your atmosphere, in other words whatever you think in your mind or speak with your mouth that is what the outcome will be. If you think negatively about your situation you will have a negative outcome. – the bibles states in **Proverbs 23:7** For as he thinketh in his heart, so is he..... We have to get into the habit of being positive and thinking positive. **Philippians 4:8** Finally, brethren, whatsoever things are true, whatsoever things are honest, whatsoever things are just, whatsoever things are pure, whatsoever things are lovely, whatsoever things are of good report; if there be any virtue, and if there be any praise, think on these things.

Ask God to purify your mind. It is so easy to lose focus especially when you are going through a battle. In my situations, I could have lost my mind and gave up being diagnosed with cancer two times in the same year. I had to ask God on numerous occasions to purify my mind while undergoing chemotherapy, radiation and the series of tests after tests. But I maintained my position and kept the faith. I began to focus on the spiritual nature of my battles and took it as an opportunity to help others. I also began to focus on the end result of my battle, I will be healed; I knew that victory was coming.

As I am writing this I began to think about a famous actor/comedian who seemed to have everything, happiness, money, fame, family, etc and yet something was missing. He became depressed over a period of time and in a moment of despair took his own life. How upsetting and disturbing this was to me. It was heartbreaking to hear of such tragedy especially someone who appeared to be so powerful but yet powerless. He could make everyone laugh around him but yet could not laugh himself. You see money and fame does not bring happiness.  How many of us are faking it?  We are walking around like everything is okay, walking as if our stuff is together and yet we are unhappy.  Now is a good time to self-exam yourself and purify your mind.  I know it is easier said than done but I want to let you know that God is a mind regulator.  He can heal you right where you hurt. He can bring peace to your mind and peace to your situation.  Why not trust Him?  I encourage you if you have tried everything and everything has failed try Jesus; He never fails.

I can write on and on about the goodness of God but let me get back to the requirements.  Another requirement to having faith in God is to

- **Visualize the Answer to your Prayers** – Prayer is the God-given tool to strengthen your
Faith and trust in Him, (Matthew 21:22)

Prayer is essential in so many matters.  You will be surprised at what God can do when you pray.  Let me explain Prayer - Prayer is conversation with God; the intercourse of the soul with God; your words connecting to the heart of God.  You may reach a point where you are going through a rough time and can't even speak; you can't seem to get the words together, I want to let you know that God understands your moans, your groans and the very tear that rolls down your cheek. Hallelujah!!

My husband is an avid do-it-yourselfer. He works on projects around the house and has been and is involved in several projects at our church.  He is a great hands-on kind of guy.  If he can't fix it, he will you-tube it and will learn how to do it.  He can repair something that is broke or build something that we may need.  He always involves our sons in his projects and has them pass him the tools that he may need from his tool case. He ensures that the boys familiarize themselves with the tools and always says that the right tools make the difference. Prayer is similar to tools. Like the right tools makes the difference so does prayer. Praying enables us to work with God. It is good to fall on your knees or do like I do sometimes I walk down the street and have a one on one conversation with God. Verbalizing how we feel to God in prayer gives us a measure of relief. Therefore let it out; He will listen to your every word.

It is fair to say that we can categorize prayer in two groups 1) one in which we ask God for something and/or 2) in which we tell Him something. Many times when we pray we are asking God for something, "Lord I need a financial blessing", "I need to be healed", "I need, I need, I need......" Other times we do not tell Him enough "Lord I appreciate you", "I praise you", "Lord do you see what is happening to me, to my family" and so on and so forth. Whichever category you fall into, our prayers, our conversations with God are our verbal tools that we use to get things done. Let me interject here and say that God does not always grant every one of our request just because we ask. Sometimes we make foolish petitions. Thank God He understands our situations and gives us what is best for us. I encourage you to pray.

After we pray and give our situations over to God we should:

- **Walk in Victory** – Walk as though it's only a matter of time before you receive your VICTORY. (I Corinthians 15:57). Walk in pride, walk with stride, hold your head up, it's going to get better you'll see.

**The Key to Victory**

- **Prayer** – Equip yourselves (Matthew 21:22) Explained in Visualize your answered prayer

- **Praise** – Praise your way to victory

As a parent when my sons do something good I applaud them with praise. Sometimes before they even do it I begin to praise them. It builds up their character and self-esteem. When we want God to do something for us we need to give Him praise even before He does it. God loves for us to express our appreciation and gratitude to Him just like our children. The particular aspects of God's character in which He was praised in the scriptures include His, goodness, loyalty, love, kindness, faithfulness, wisdom, trustfulness, omnipresence and compassion; we too can praise Him for those very things. So begin to praise God right where you are for what He is about to do. We need to give Him a just because praise. In our everyday lives we need to begin to give God a just because PRAISE.

- **Fasting** - Fasting let's God know that what you have asked Him for you really want it.

What is fasting? According to ıdictionary.com it defines fasting as abstain from all or some kinds of food or drink, especially as a religious observance.

Fasting and praying in some instances go hand and hand and can be found in numerous passages of scripture. The purpose of fasting is spiritual – it is to devote the time you spend eating and drinking to God; a more pressing need to devote your entire being to God rather than fueling your body. Oftentimes people fast for various reasons, some do it to cleanse the body of impurities while others do it for mental purposes, to clear their minds so that they can concentrate a little better. Fasting expresses how strongly we are willing to forego eating to pray and devote all to God. It shows how strongly we feel about what we are praying about. Some situations may require us to fast and pray; as mentioned in Mark 9:29; And He said unto them, This kind can come forth by nothing, but by prayer and fasting. Fasting and praying enables us to concentrate in prayer and to call on God with unusual intensity to answer.

The desire to have your prayers answered through fasting and praying is what moves God. If your child asks you for something more than likely you will consider giving it to them because you love your child and want to give them what they asked for within reason. However your decision to give, delay giving or withhold what they have asked for depends on many factors. If your child is persistent in asking for the same thing you know that it is important to them. This will incline you to further grant the request if it is in the best interest of your child. Similarly fasting demonstrates to God how much we want what we ask Him for. It will not force Him to act swifter to grant our petition but will incline Him to do more if we fast.

1Dictionary.com

- **Positiveness** – Do not allow negativity into your spirit

Positive defined in the Webster's II New College Dictionary is marked by or exhibiting certainty, acceptance or affirmation; admitting of no doubt. How many times have your mind gone in the wrong direction and you begin to doubt God and what He can do; Countless times. I have been there myself and had to encourage myself. I had to replace that negative thought or feeling with positivity. I had to look at the end result of my situation and move forward. Once I got my mind back on the right track, I could see victory. Be sure to ask God to keep your mind because Satan's desire is to get your mind, if he could get your mind he can toy with you. Keep a positive outlook regardless of what it looks like, victory is coming. God is perfecting your faith through the opportunities that come with your challenges. Your responses to the difficult challenges will define your level and strength of your trust in God. I encourage you to persevere and move through your challenges with faith and grace. Be strong, be courageous, be patient, and be positive.

## James 1:2-4

**[2] My brethren, count it all joy when ye fall into divers temptations; [3] Knowing this, that the trying of your faith worketh patience. [4] But let patience have her perfect work, that ye may be perfect and entire, wanting nothing.**

If you do your part God will do His. My prayer is that you will learn to trust God completely. The secret to victory is to dwell on God's ability to handle your situations. Live as if your request has been granted. You will never be the same again.

• **Forgiveness** – Let go of past hurts and experiences. Wow, this is a hard one even for me!! Forgiveness could mean giving up your right to hurt someone that hurt you. So many times people have done things to hurt you and we think of all the things we can do to get back at them. But at the end of the day is it worth it!! It is impossible to live on this earth without getting hurt, offended, misunderstood, lied to, lied on and/or rejected. Such is life! We need to get over it, I know it's hard but in order to obtain complete victory we have to let some things go.

The Webster II New College Dictionary defines Forgiveness as the following: to excuse for a fault or offense. When you wrong someone or someone wrongs you it is good to forgive so that the relationship can be restored. It is important to say that forgiveness is not granted because the person deserves to be forgiven; instead it is an act of love, mercy and grace. It is only God's mercy and grace that He died for our sins; He didn't have to do it but he showed us an act of love by hanging on the cross for you and for me. He was hung and stretched wide on the cross; goodness in one hand, mercy on the other as they nailed His hands to the cross. He had a heart of love for us. If we follow in God's steps we too can forgive. Just because we forgive someone doesn't mean that we will put ourselves back into a harmful situation or that we approve of the person's wrong behavior. It simply means that we are released from the wrong that was committed. We have to forgive because God forgave us. (Ephesians 4:31-32) If God had not forgiven us where would we be, we would be in a mess!! I will admit there are times and times will occur when we don't feel like forgiving or we don't want to forgive; it is much easier to act on the hurt we feel rather than disconnecting ourselves from the hurt. Not forgiving others can bring on bitterness and stress. In order to free ourselves physically, spiritually, emotionally we must forgive. Forgiveness is an act of our own personal will; it is a direct submission to God's will, trusting God to be emotionally healed.

## Matthew 6:14-15
**For if you forgive other people when they sin against you, your heavenly Father will also forgive you. But if you do not forgive others their sins, your Father will not forgive your sins.**

As I write this I am looking in the mirror of my soul. I too have had a difficult time with forgiving. I found myself harboring over things that people have done or said to me and have had a difficult time trying to forgive. But when my back was up against a wall and I was placed in a situation where I had to pray, it was then God began to deal with me and I realized that I had to let go of the hurt and disappointments. I had to free myself in order to be myself. Once you really break free and mean it from your heart you will be released of the hurt, the pain. It is then you can be free. Once I let it go I felt such a burden lift off of my shoulder and I promised myself that I will not be entangled in it again. I say to you let it go; set your soul free. **"Break Free".** Once you are free be not entangled again with the yoke of bondage and don't allow the enemy to entangle you again.

## Galatians 5:1
**Stand fast therefore in the liberty wherewith Christ hath made us free, and be not entangled again with the yoke of bondage.**

### How Do I Forgive
When every fiber of your being tells you not to forgive, how does one forgive?

- Romans 5:6 states for when we were yet without strength, in due time Christ died for the
  ungodly. Remind yourself that God forgave you; he died so that you can live; if he can forgive you and hang on the cross for you, for me we too can forgive. I know it's hard but it can be done!
- Forgive not for the person that hurt you but for yourself. It enables you to have peace of
  mind.
- It's so much easier to forgive than to hang on to so much anger, hurt and betrayal.
- Do not keep dwelling on the past or the bad thing that happened; when you let go of it,
  You get over the anger/bitterness that you felt and it clears the path for forgiveness!
- The harder it is to forgive someone else, the more you are held accountable.
- Learn to forgive yourself and forgiving others more than likely will be easier.

- Forgiveness comes easy when you know that what people say or do is about them, it's
  not about you.
- Forgiveness takes away the power the other person continues to wield in your life.

- Allow God to heal the brokenness; the more you allow Him to heal the better your life
  will become. It may not be instant. It may take time but it's worth the relief, the forgiveness and the peace you feel.
- Don't let guilt wreak havoc on your body, mind and soul. You don't have to live with the
  guilt any longer. Let it all go; it's not worth it!

The few tips on how to forgive mentioned above is what helped me to forgive and move on. I promised myself that I will not get back in that situation again. Once I forgave I stayed away from the one that caused the pain in the first place that was for my own sanity. I had to pray on myself and had to rebuke the negative thoughts that tried to cloud my mind. Every now and again I have to rebuke myself too!! I had to let the pain go, let the disappointment go, let the confusion go, just let it go, let it go, let it go. I began to focus more on me and less on the pain. Once I was able to really break free of my pain, my worship was different, my thoughts were different, my outlook was different and my healing was on its way. Hallelujah!!!

**Remember:** The Formula to obtain total victory and healing is:

**Prayer + Praise + Fasting + Having a Positive Attitude + Forgiveness = TOTAL VICORY**

As I conclude with this chapter my journey of faith, strength, and endurance, believing in the promise of God and trusting in God was an enlightening experience. I learned a great deal about me and the power I had within. When I began this journey my focus was on why I had to go through the situation of being diagnosed with cancer but as I continued the course my views were different. Just because one is diagnosed with a condition does not necessary mean you are going to die with the diagnosis. I began to view it in the eyes of God and looked at the end result; the end result resulting in victory. I invite you to reach deep within yourselves and awake the spiritual being in you so that you too can obtain victory. Otherwise you may become overwhelmed by your circumstances and never obtain total victory. I have mentioned throughout this book the power of positive thinking and taking God at His Word. I encourage you to allow God's Word to come alive in your lives. I am no different than you and because of human nature you will have negative thoughts and at some point the devil will make sure you see and hear about all the bad that has happened to everyone who was diagnosed with your condition. On many occasions I've had people discuss with me people who have died with breast and colon cancer; like I really wanted to hear that!! It took some time for me to dismiss the thoughts from my mind and not allow what I've seen or heard steer me away from my stand in faith. I had to learn to encourage myself daily and say these words, "I will live and not die".

## Ezekiel 18:28
**Because he considereth, and turneth away from all his transgressions that he hath committed, he shall surely live, he shall not die.**

## A Test of Faith

I will admit that when I first heard the word cancer come out of the mouth of the doctor my faith was indeed shaken. But as the days progressed I prayed and spoke God's Word into my spirit being. I can see how it is easy to give up than to fight, but if God blesses you with breath in your body, you need to fight! In that fight you have to believe that God can heal and bring you out of the situation you are in. Mark 11:24 discusses the power of asking God for something when you pray. You must not only ask but believe that you will receive it. Like that of a parent when you ask your parents for something, you ask with the expectation that you will receive what you have asked for as long as it is within reason. The same when asking God, ask with expectation that you will receive that which you have asked. God is not like man, you can ask for those things which are not within reason that is the kind of God He is. He can give you your desire even if it is out of man's reach.

## Mark 11:24

**Therefore I say unto you, What things soever ye desire, when ye pray, believe that ye receive them, and ye shall have them.**

Many of you do not understand faith and how it works. Let me reiterate you have to believe that what you ask for you will receive it the moment you speak it out of your mouth. What is the use of praying and asking if you are not going to believe? The Word says **believe that ye receive them, and ye shall have them** – that's faith in action. Set faith in motion and watch God work.

### A Test of Strength
My strength in God was tested but after it was all said and done I gained strength I never knew I had. Because of the strength I gained I was able to endure; endure the chemotherapy treatments, endure the side effects of chemotherapy, the hair loss, loss of appetite nauseated feelings, the weakness. But during the treatments God was merciful to me, before the chemotherapy treatments every single one of my blood tests which the lab would take to ensure that my body was handling the treatments adequately came back fine. I thank God that in almost a year and a half of treatment I never had to postpone any of the treatments. My oncologist would always say "Your blood levels are good". Nevertheless the treatments were very hard but I had to do what I had to do. God enabled me to endure the radiation treatments. I constantly prayed and blessed God at all times for all things. I would often repeat Philippians 4:13 to myself, I can do all things through Christ who strengthens me.

## Philippians 4:13
## I can do all things through Christ which strengtheneth me.

### The Courage to Endure
I know it was God and His Word that helped me make it through the treatments as well as I did. I came to the realization that my endurance was being built while I was going through this test. Some tests are designed to build you up and take you to another level or plateau. I work for the City of New York and many times promotional tests are given to employees so that they have the opportunity to be promoted. It is up to the employee to take advantage of the test. The same concept applies in the spiritual realm you

have to do something to get something. I had take the test in order to be promoted to the next level or plateau.

Now that I have endured I had to believe the promises of God. I prayed for healing, I endured and now I had to believe the promises of God. His Word declares in II Corinthians 1:20 that all the promises of God in Him are yea, and in Him Amen. God put the period at the end of the sentence when it was stated: **For all the promises of God in him are yea, and in him Amen.** When you have finish praying you end with amen; that is the end. The end of that chapter in your life of suffering and circumstances has already been written it is up to you to follow the course all the way to the end. Amen!

## II Corinthians 1:20
**For all the promises of God in him are yea, and in him Amen, unto the glory of God by us.**

### Who Can We Trust
My faith, my strength, my courage to endure while believing the promise of God played a role in my victory. And as I continued my journey trust was a huge factor on my road to healing. I have learned to put my total trust in God each day. I had to trust God for healing and the hands of the physicians who were working on my behalf. I know it may sound a little redundant trusting God and trusting the physicians but it is not. I had to trust the physicians that God placed in my path for the healing to manifest. Because of God and the efforts from the physicians I was able to break free of me and allow God to work in me and through me. I was able to break free from negativity and allow positive thoughts to take over. I was able to break

free of past hurtful experiences so that God can work freely. I've mentioned on several occasions that it was not easy to do all of the things mentioned above but it can be done. You have to renew your mind each day as stated in Romans 12:2.

### Romans 12:2
**And be not conformed to this world: but be ye transformed by the renewing of your mind, that ye may prove what is that good, and acceptable, and perfect, will of God.**

As I close this chapter I want to encourage you. If you have heard a negative report from your doctor and are waiting for healing seek God, except the help from your doctor and Trust God to work through the doctors to get you all the help and assistance you may need. What you do not need to be doing is doing absolutely nothing while waiting and consoling yourself with a hope of a miracle. Some of you may think that if you consult a physician or follow his or her advice you are not operating in faith. I beg to differ; if your faith was not strong enough to keep an attack on your body from coming against you in the first place, how are you going to believe for the attack to just disappear? Food for thought!!!

Please I invoke you to have your yearly physicals, not only have them but follow-up on the results. If anything arises ask God to place you in the best doctor's care and follow the advice of your physician. Importantly pray, stay positive and allow God to work in you and through you. I am writing from experience not hearsay, I tell you it works. God has no respect of persons what He has done for me He can do for you.

## Romans 2:11
### For there is no respect of persons with God.

In the beginning of this book a question was asked: *Is there anything too hard for God?*

My reply **"<u>NO</u>"** there is NOTHING TOO HARD FOR GOD.

### My Prayer for You

Lord I ask that all those who have read this book have gained insight of you. *I pray that whatever they are facing or will be placed in their lives that the words of this book will come alive for them. Lord I pray that you would bless each person today and everyday. Lord I ask that you would restore health and renew minds. I know that there is nothing too hard for you to do.*

## Psalm 19:14
### Let the words of my mouth, and the meditation of my heart, be acceptable in thy sight, O LORD, my strength, and my redeemer.

## Numbers 6:26
### The Lord lift up his countenance upon thee, and give thee peace.

# *Words of Encouragement*

Joshua 1:9
Have not I commanded thee? Be strong and of a
good courage; be not afraid, neither be thou
dismayed: for the Lord thy God is with thee
whithersoever thou goest.

It is always amazing when you receive a word of encouragement when you need it the most. After being diagnosed with cancer or any other disease it is easy for one to become discouraged and or want to give up. When I came to work this particular day (Jan. 27, 2014) I was feeling a little down and wouldn't you know it, a word came just when I needed it. The first three words captured my attention "Listen to Me". I had to open my mind and my heart and adhere to the words that were written just for me. As I approached the end of this book the words captioned below are crystal clear: Those things you have endured have made you stronger where I am able to tell you that you too can be victorious.

## THE TRUMPET by BILL BURNS

Listen to me. I know what you have been through. I know the harshness of the past season that you have had to endure. I know the reality of that, but please understand that it was for your benefit; the benefit of strength of your trust in me. Those things that you have endured and gone through have made you stronger if you believe they have. And, as you come out into a new season you will find the strength I have given you will become a reality. It stretched you and caused you to walk with greater dignity, greater revelation, greater focus than ever before. This new reality will benefit you in the season that is now unfolding before you. So leave those things in My hand. The things you endured will now become your ornaments—they tell the world, tell the enemy you have been through something and you have come out victoriously on this side of it. This day, see yourself as victorious, says the Lord.

## SMALL STRAWS IN A SOFT WIND By MARSHA BURNS:

Enhance the quality of your life by adding more spiritual content. I have not called you to be paupers in My kingdom, but to feed sumptuously on My Word and to walk on the path that leads to abundant life. Many of My people, however live like there is not enough to go around. Continually seek My face and let My Word and My purposes abound in, around and through you, says the Lord. John 10:10 The theif does not come except ot steal, and to kill, and to destroy. I have come that they may have life, and that they may have it more abundantly.

## ₁Faith Tabernacle
## January 27, 2014

Wow what a word, I needed to hear!

Reference:1Faith Tabernacle – The Trumpet by Bill Burns/Marsha Burns

# Doctor's Notes

Luke 2:46
And it came to pass, that after three days they found him in the temple, sitting in the midst of the **doctor**s, both hearing them, and asking them questions.

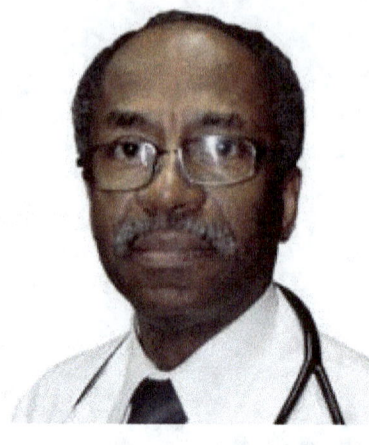

*A Message from Dr. Arpel Nicoleau*
**Queensvillage Medical**

I have known Sharon professionally since April 1995. As her medical doctor I have treated her for hypertension and allergies.

In June 2013 she was diagnosed with breast cancer, a much more serious condition. She underwent a lumpectomy in September 2013 followed by chemotherapy and radiation. Several factors stood out in Sharon's case. A lot of people procrastinate after learning of an "abnormal mammogram" leading to a delay in diagnosis. Sharon kept all her appointments and tackled the problem head on. She did not rely solely on us physician (she was uniquely cooperative however) but read on all aspect of her disease and became very familiar with the medical jargon. She learned what staging entailed and learned about Hormone Receptors for example.

Why did Sharon do so well with little discomfort from her chemotherapy and radiation compare with other patient with the same disease burden? The relationship between mind and body has been known for a long time. Sir William Osler, the great British clinician even said "it is more important to know what patient has a disease than what disease a patient has". Sharon's spiritual side was crucial in molding her attitude to adversities. In the bible the writer says "I can do all things through Christ who strengthen me."(Philippians 4:13). Sharon could have made the same statement.

She is now officially cancer free as of January 2015, meaning that there is no residual cancer by physical examination and by biological markers. I believe the outstanding result of her treatment is not due to solely to the skills of her medical team (we in the medical filed can have huge egos!) But also to her spiritual beliefs and mental attitude. This in turn leads to a greater cooperation with her physicians, provides resilience and determination .I think her story will empower a lot of people who may the same challenges.

92-04 Springfield Boulevard * Queensvillage, NY 11428 * T. (718) 465-3040 * F. (718) 464-9063

# From
## The
### Desk of
#### Dr. Malvina Fulman

As a doctor we come across many different kinds of people every day. Many of the people I encounter have different prognosis and diagnosis. Sharon Robinson came to me as a referral from her surgeon when she was diagnosed with Colon Cancer. Upon seeing her she was very concerned as any patient would be about her diagnosis. As I sat and reviewed the pathology report with both her and her husband, they were very tentative to what I was saying. I can remember telling her that because her right colon was removed and reconstructed I was happy to report that she would not need chemotherapy or radiation. Her face just lit up. She had a question about if the colon cancer would return and as her doctor had to state the facts that anything is possible although the chances were slim. I informed her that she would be under observation for a few years and would have a colonoscopy every six months. If things are looking well she would then have a colonoscopy once a year still with close observation.

I then saw Sharon Robinson approximately six (6) months later with a different diagnosis. She was diagnosed with cancer in the right breast. Upon seeing her and her husband once again they both were concerned and had many questions. After her lumpectomy, I had the job of letting her know that it was my recommendation that she undergo chemotherapy and radiation because her HER2 receptors cells had more than normal which could cause the cancer cells to grow and divide rapidly if the cancer returned. In order to get a head start on this to help to prevent the cancer from returning, it was a good idea for her to undergo chemotherapy and radiation. It would help narrow the chances of the cancer returning. Sharon's state of mind was remarkable. Everyone handles situations differently whether you are an optimist or a pessimist. I found Sharon to be an optimist she stood strongly on her beliefs and did not allow the pressure of her diagnosis and or undergoing chemotherapy and radiation get her down. Every time she entered my office for chemotherapy she looked great even when she was not feeling her best, was in good spirits and was very spiritual. I believe that it was her faith that got her through her ordeals along with the assistance of the doctors. She was a great patient who not only kept her appointments but asked many questions.

When she expressed to me that she was writing a book of her experiences with colon and breast cancer and asked me to write something on her behalf I jumped at the opportunity to help her inspire others. She has inspired so many.

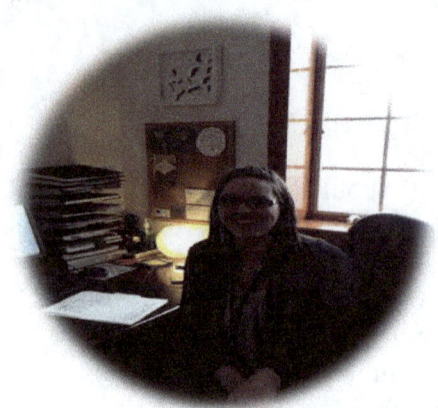

## From the Desk of
## Caroline Rung Elsas,
## Genetic Counselor

When Sharon came for her first genetic counseling appointment, she was glowing. She greeted me with a big smile and a friendly hello. We sat down and she told me a bit about her story, how she had battled two cancers in the same year while being a wife, raising two children and working. I found myself inspired by her positive outlook and bright spirit despite all of the difficulties she was facing. After a discussion about genetic testing, Sharon decided to proceed with the test. She said she wanted the information in case it would help guide future management for her and her two sons. We agreed to meet a few weeks later when the results were ready.

When Sharon returned, I revealed the findings to her. Sharon was found to carry a variant of uncertain significance in the *PMS2* gene. This gene is implicated in colon, uterine, and other cancers. There is also some evidence to suggest that it may be involved with breast cancer but this has not been confirmed. It was explained that the lab does not yet have enough information about this genetic change to classify it as deleterious or benign. It is unclear at this time whether the change contributes to an increased risk for cancer. Sharon's current medical management will not be changed and other family members will not be tested for this change since its significance is unclear and the results are not informative of risk. I explained that it would be beneficial for Sharon to follow up with me yearly, since the result will be reclassified as a positive or negative after more data is available. If one day we find that this variant contributes to a risk for cancer, Sharon will either be monitored closely for uterine cancer or have a preventive hysterectomy. We would also recommend increased screening for other cancer types which are linked to the *PMS2* gene.

For some patients, uninformative results can be anxiety provoking. In addition to everything they have already been through, it may add to feelings of uncertainty about their future. It was interesting that before Sharon left my office, she told me how I really made her feel at ease about the genetic counseling and testing process. I would have thought that she may leave more anxious than she had come, especially given her inconclusive result. Sharon seemed to be at ease about the genetic counselor process and at peace with the uncertain result. Her strength in dealing with her medical situation was amazing.

For further information you can contact the NSGC.org website and the find a genetic counselor function (http://nsgc.org/p/cm/ld/fid=164) to find a counselor in your area.

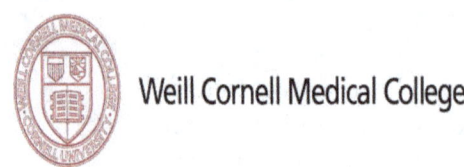

**Leonard A. Farber, MD**
Clinical Director and Associate Professor
New York Presbyterian/Weill Cornell Medical College
Fax: 917.210.3285

**Re: Sharon Robinson**

**History:**
47-year old Pre-Menopausal Female with a history of colon cancer and recent diagnosis of breast cancer.

5/24/13: Mammogram. Abnormal mammogram, requires additional view.
6/5/13: Spot compression mammogram. 10 mm cyst with debris vs. solid nodule at 10:00 axis in the right breast.
6/19/13: Stereotactic biopsy. Positive for IDC, poorly differentiated 12 mm in greatest dimension in the right breast.
7/19/13: MRI. 0.8 cm enhancing enhancing nodule in the right breast 8:00 axis consistent with malignant diagnosis, 1 cm
enhancement lesion in the right breast 9:00 axis corresponding with mammographic nodule, Left breast negative.
7/30/13: Ultrasound. 8:00 axis of the right breast corresponds with prior biopsied malignancy and 8:30, 0.9 cm nodule; biopsy recommended.
8/14/13: Biopsy. Benign pathology of the 8:30, 1 cm ovoid lesion in the right breast.
9/20/13: Lumpectomy with SLN biopsy. 2 foci IDC, poorly differentiated (Nottingham: 3+3+3), spans 0.6 cm and 1.2 cm.
Extensive high grade DCIS, Grade III (solid and cribriform

types with comedo necrosis), microcalcification present with DCIS. Both IDC and DCIS ER/PR+, Her2 3+; both have approximately 40% KI67 proliferative indices. SLN (0,1), LN (0,1), IDC margin 2.2 mm, DCIS margin <1 mm.
10/7/13: CT Chest. No axillary, hilar, or mediastinal lymphadenopathy.
10/13/13: BRCA 1/2. Negative.

She underwent adjuvant ACT chemotherapy followed by Herceptin and presented for treatment with radiation therapy.

Sharon underwent radiation therapy to the right breast from 5.12.2014-7.17.2014. Treatments were given daily, 5 days a week, Monday through Friday. Her treatment took approximate 3 to 5 minutes and she was in the office of a total of 20-25 minutes.

Sharon was an absolute delight to have in the office. She came in every day with a smile and warmth and that was not only palpable, but contagious. She left every day with that same smile. She completed all her treatments on time and was diligent about making her appointments as scheduled.

In Sharon's clinical setting radiation is a part of her required breast conservation treatment. It is an equivalent outcome procedure to a mastectomy with her surgery and chemotherapy and she was able to preserve her breast by not omitting the treatment modalities. Radiation in the post-lumpectomy setting reduces the overall risk of her cancer coming back and can significantly impact on her survival. Numerous published studies have demonstrated that and therefore radiation was considered to be an essential component of her treatment. Sharon recognized the data and need for using the different modalities to treat her. She embraced the treatment, and was determined to see it through in the special way that makes her the way she is.

Sharon will be followed routinely by her physicians with physical examination, mammograms, and other required imaging studies. My overall opinion is that she will do quite well.

I am delighted to have had the opportunity to be a part of Sharon's care and to have gotten to know her as a person beyond her just being my patient.

# The Farber Center Staff

**Me & Dr. Leonard Farber**    **The Radiation Technicians**

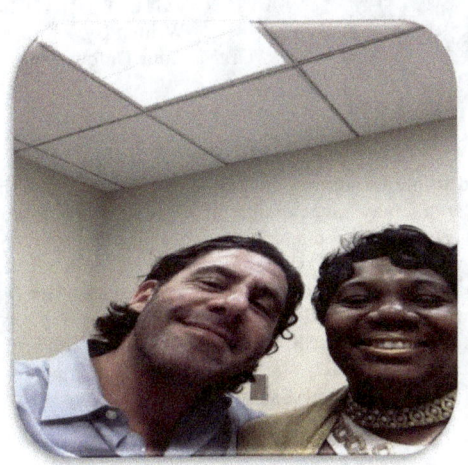
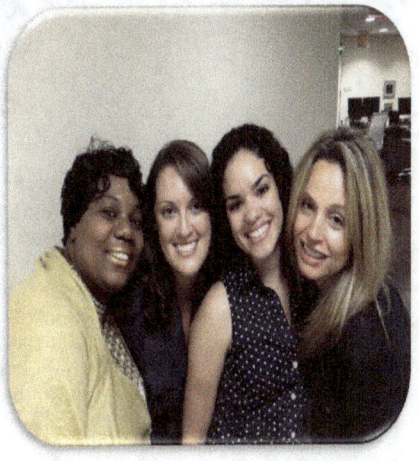

**The Doctor's Assistant**          **The Office Manager**

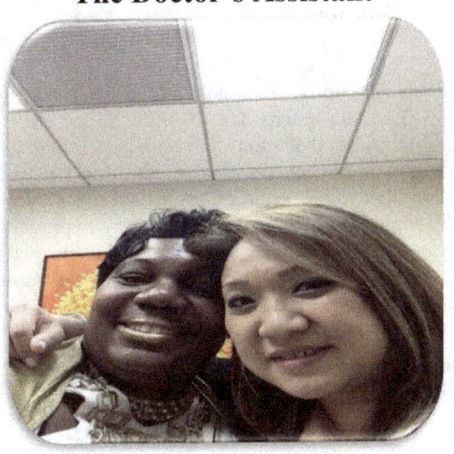
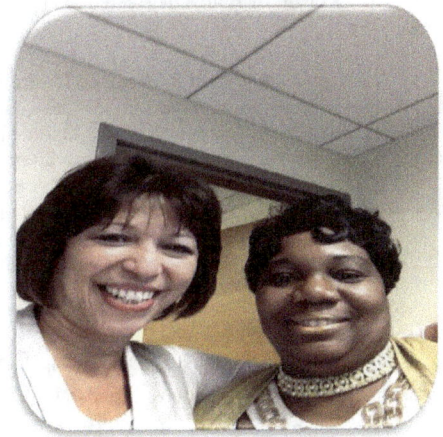

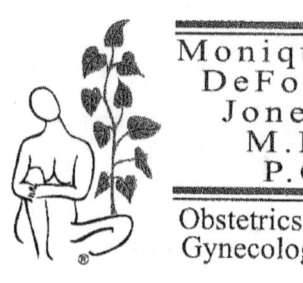

# Monique DeFour Jones, M.D. P.C.
## Obstetrics & Gynecology

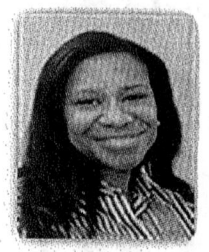

**A PREGNANT WARRIOR**
Written By:
Dr. Monique Defour-Jones

**SHARON ROBINSON** was referred to me by her internist after she was told that she had begun to dilate in the first trimester and may have possibly miscarried. At this point, this was her sixth pregnancy and she was advanced maternal age (over the age of thirty-five) and had loss the five other pregnancies; one of which was in the second trimester. She also had a history of chronic hypertension and fibroids. When I saw Sharon she was quite tearful because of the previous miscarriages. All she wanted was to carry full term and have a healthy baby. She had already begun bleeding prior to her ninth week of the pregnancy. After all of her testing was completed she was found to have cervical dilation and bleeding. An ultrasound was done reveal a sub-chorionic hematoma which was the cause of her bleeding.

Sharon and her husband were counseled extensively regarding the risk of another pregnancy loss. I explained to them that I would place a cerclage (stitch), but that that was not a 100% guarantee. I explained that we would have to leave this pregnancy in God's hands. She was so nervous about another loss but she stated that God would take care of it all. At twelve (12) weeks the cerclage was placed and she was placed on bed rest.

Although on bed rest, she continued to dilate her cervix. With close fetal surveillance, her membrane started to funnel (come down) to the stitch. On 5/13/2002, Sharon was admitted to North Shore University Hospital in Manhasset at 24 weeks gestation due to cervical incompetence and dilation through the cerclage. She was placed on strict bed rest and in trendelenburg (the bed upside down). She handled being laid upside down very well. I can remember her husband bringing from home their computer and printer as I watched in amazement her do a wedding program from the bed. She had unbelievable strength. This was a very difficult time for Sharon because this is a very critical age for the baby. She was given an injection of steroids to help accelerate fetal lung maturity. She was on antihypertensive medication to control her blood pressure.

During her ten week stay at the hospital, she was found to have contraction (preterm labor) and required medication to stop the contractions. She also developed gestational diabetes and this required a special diet and glucose monitoring. Her baby also had to have special monitoring called a non stress test and biophysical profile. Sharon always had a positive outlook on her pregnancy and I believe that her strong faith in God made a

444 Community Drive • Suite 201 • Manhasset, N.Y. 11030 • T: (516) 869-8071 • F: (516) 869-801⁹

marked difference in her successful outcome. Don't get me wrong there were some days that Sharon was a little anxious but overall she remained compliant and calm.

Sharon always wanted to be kept abreast of what was going on with the pregnancy and I would explain that would take each day as it comes and thank God for another day that the baby remained in her uterus. She was discharged home in July at 34 ½ weeks.

On August 8, Sharon ruptured membranes at approximately 11:30p.m. She was 36 ½ weeks. She was three and a half weeks early. Her cerclage was removed and she delivered a live infant Male, 5 pounds 10 ounces on August 9th at 7:56pm with excellent Apgar scores.

Sharon was a great patient. Her strong faith in God, her positive attitude and her belief in me as her doctor got her where she is today. She was compliant with what was asked of her; the strict bed rest, the glycemic monitoring for her diabetes and taking her medication for her blood pressure and the necessary testing for the fetal surveillance. I could not have asked for a better patient and as a result she had a beautiful and victorious outcome. She and her husband were elated to get their baby home.

Sharon had a subsequent pregnancy in 2004. She had similar medical and obstetrical issues and again required a cerclage and best rest. With her strong faith in God, she went on to delivery another male infant 6 pounds 2 ounces on 5/22/2004.

I was overjoyed to be a part of her victorious story. As doctors we are faced with difficult decisions every day and it is great when we can share success stories and this is one of them.

# *Support*

Acts 20:35
I have shewed you all things, how that so labouring ye ought to **support** the weak, and to remember the words of the Lord Jesus, how he said, It is more blessed to give than to receive.

# Supporter Page

This page is dedicated to all those who called to encourage me, came to see me whether in the hospital or at home and those who called who did not know what was going on with me but wanted to have prayer with me via of the telephone as well as those who did not know what was going on but prayed for me when they did not see me. I thank you for your love and support. Thank you to Bishop Wright & Mother Wright for coming to administer communion to me. Thank you to my Greater Refuge Church Family who prayed for me and those of you who asked my husband for me; he gave me every message. Thank you for your support.

## Family
Nelleen Underwood
Pearl Woods-Robinson
Steavenson & Martha Hendricks
Bishop Walter Lee Jackson & Mother Margaret Jackson
Brenda Jackson
Mr. Nathan & Dr. Sheryl Johnson
Charles Robinson & Family

## Church Family
Bishop Charles E. Wright & Mother Faye Wright
Bishop Wilbur L. Jones & Mother Sandra Jones
Bishop William Wilkins & Lady Sara Wilkins
Elder Michael Bouie & Lady Janean Bouie
Elder Richard Lord & Lady Sheila Lord
Elder Reginald Brown & Lady Natalie Brown
Laurence Rivers & Charlene Rivers
Evangelist Helen McNeal
Mother Julia Jenkins
Mother Mable Kennon

Missionary Gladys Leonard
Missionary Sadie Hudson
Dr. Frances L. Hamilton
Deloris Moore
Gwendolyn Gainer
Greta Anderson
Joy Middleton
Geraldine Spigner
Carly Bell
Gloria Phipps
Van Jay McDuffy
Keisha Swain-Andrews
Celeste Green
Michele Brown
Carol Williams
Patricia Lindsay
**And the Entire Greater Refuge Temple Family and Beulah Church of Christ Family**

## Co-Workers
Susan Haskell
Francine Mallozzi
Regina Miller
Christopher Cesarani
Meryl Jones
Rhodeisa Humphrey
Beatrice Parker
Yvonne Harris
Nichelle Desousa
Rosemarie Thompson-Brown
Kara Moyston
Karen Alexander
Rosita Primus
Stracy Stewart
Jacqueline Roberts
Denice Williams

## <u>Other Friends</u>
Ethel Cooks
Karla Cooks
Janice Wallace
Rachel Berry

# Informative Information

Daniel 9:22
And he **inform**ed me, and talked with me, and said, O Daniel, I am now come forth to give thee skill and understanding.

# Informative Information

## ₁What is Colon Cancer

Colon cancer is a type of cancer that develops in the large intestine. Our colons are about 6 feet long and allow waste to travel from the small intestine to the rectum. Like other organs in our body, the colon is vulnerable to many diseases and conditions, like cancer.

### Colon Cancer Causes and Risk Factors

At this time, we can't exactly pinpoint what causes colon cancer, but we do know what may make our risk of developing colon cancer greater. Risk factors for colon cancer include:

- **Age.** As you age, your risk for developing colon cancer increases. Colon cancer most often occurs in adults over the age of 50, but it can still occur in younger adults.

- **Race and Ethnicity.** African Americans are at a greater risk of developing colon cancer than any other race, although it is unclear why. Ashkenazi Jews (Jews of European descent) are also at high risk of developing colon cancer. Several inherited genetic mutations have been found in Ashkenazi Jews, which greatly contributes to their increased risk.

- **Family Medical History.** If you have a family history of colon cancer, you may be at a greater risk of developing the disease, too. A person does not need a family history of colon cancer to have colon cancer; it is most commonly diagnosed in those without a family history.

- **Personal Medical History.** Having polyps, small growths in the colon, puts you at risk of developing colon cancer. Seventy percent to 90% of colon cancer cases develop from polyps, and having them removed reduces your risk of colon cancer. Once removed, they can return, which makes colon cancer screening a vital part of maintaining colon health. You are also more at risk if you suffer from inflammatory bowel disease (IBD), a condition that causes the colon to become inflamed.

- **Genetics.** Two inherited syndromes commonly associated with a marked increase in colon cancer risk are familial adenomatous polyposis (FAP) and hereditary non-polyposis colon cancer(HNPCC). About 5% of colon cancer cases are caused by a inherited syndrome. Peutz-Jeghers syndrome is a much less common syndrome that is also associated with colon cancer.

- **Other Identified Risk Factors:** There are many other identified colon cancer risk factors, such as smoking cigarettes, consuming alcohol, level of physical activity, obesity, and diagnosis of type 2 diabetes.

## Colon Cancer Symptoms

In the early stages, colon cancer usually doesn't have symptoms. As the disease progresses, which can take years, symptoms include:

- Blood in stool
- Persistent constipation, diarrhea, or other bowel changes
- Thinner stools
- Unexplained weight loss

- Abdominal pain and discomfort- generally feeling full, bloated, or cramping
- Abdominal tenderness or pain
- Fatigue

These colon cancer symptoms are not unique and can also be symptoms of many other conditions.

## Colon Cancer Screening

Several screening methods are highly effective at detecting colon cancer. Colon cancer screening tests include:

- **Colonoscopy.** A colonoscopy allows the doctor to get an in-depth view of the colon with the use of a colonoscope, a fiber optic tube that is attached to a microscopic camera that transmits live video feed to a monitor. The colonoscope is gently inserted into the anus and slowly to the colon, giving the doctor a full view of the rectum and large intestine. It is common to be nervous about a colonoscopy, so people are given a sedative prior to the procedure to aid in relaxation, and also to help the doctor complete the colonoscopy.
- **Sigmoidoscopy.** Much like a colonoscopy, a sigmoidoscopy is done with a flexible, lighted tube with an attached camera, but it is limited to only the lower part of the colon.
- **Barium Enema.** During a barium enema, a doctor inserts liquid barium into the rectum. X-rays are taken of you laying several positions. The barium allows the colon to be viewed better on X-rays.
- **Fecal Occult Blood Test.** A fecal occult blood test (FOBT) finds blood in your stool that you may not see with the naked eye or to confirm that it is actually blood in the

stool that you may have seen. You are given a special kit to collect stool samples.

For adults who are at average risk of colon cancer, it is recommended to begin screening for colon cancer at age 50. Adults who are classified at higher risk may begin screening earlier at the recommendation of their doctor. Remember that even if you are not experiencing symptoms of colon cancer, you should always follow your doctor's colon cancer screening recommendations.

## Diagnosing Colon Cancer

If a screening test reveals suspicious results, then a colon biopsy is done. A colon biopsy can be conveniently done during a colonoscopy or can also be done surgically. During a colon biopsy, small amounts of colon tissue are removed and then sent to a pathology lab to screen for evidence of cancer. If cancer is present, then the stage of colon cancer is then determined through colon cancer surgery to remove the cancer. Surrounding lymph nodes are tested and may also be removed during the surgery.

### Treatment of Colon Cancer
**Surgery:**   Most people with colon cancer will undergo some type of colon surgery. It is a common method of treatment and often accompanies another type of surgery. Types of surgery used to treat colon cancer include:

•       **Local Incision and Polypectomy:**   In early stage colon cancer, a surgeon may be able to remove cancerous tissue without actually having to make an incision in the abdomen. Special instruments are inserted into the rectum to the colon cancer the cancer is removed. If the cancer is found in a polyp, then is it referred to as a polypectomy.

**Surgical Resection:** During a surgical resection, a surgeon removes part of the colon and then the colon is reconnected. This can be achieved through an abdominal incision, or for some people, laparoscopically. Laparoscopic assisted resection is a relatively new approach of performing a resection, so a surgeon experienced in this method is needed. It is not recommended for all people, more so for those with earlier stages of colon cancer. A colon resection is also called a colectomy or segmental resection. Several types of resections are performed based on the stage of colon cancer and other factors.

**Resection and Colostomy:** When the colon is not reattached during a resection, a colostomy is an option that provides an effective way for waste material to leave the body. The end of the large intestine is brought through the abdominal wall to an opening (a stoma) in the abdomen that allows waste material to drain into a bag, called a colostomy bag. A colostomy may be temporary or permanent.

**Chemotherapy**: The organs in our body are made up of cells. Cells divide and multiply as the body needs them. When these cells continue to multiply unnecessarily, the result is a mass or growth, also called a tumor. Chemotherapy drugs work by eliminating these rapidly multiplying renegade cells. Other healthy cells multiply just as quickly, like hair follicle cells. Unfortunately, many chemotherapy drugs may not be able to discern the two, attacking healthy cells and causing side effects like hair loss.

Chemotherapy for colon cancer may be advised in those with stage 2 colon cancer and in those suffering from stages 3 and 4. Chemotherapy for colon cancer may be prescribed before or after surgery and may also be given in conjunction with radiation therapy.

**Radiation Therapy**: Radiation therapy uses certain types high energy beams of radiation to shrink tumors or eliminate cancer cells. Radiation therapy works by damaging a cancer cell's DNA, making it unable to multiply. Although radiation therapy can damage nearby healthy cells, cancer cells are highly sensitive to radiation and typically die when treated. Healthy cells that are damaged during radiation are resilient and are often able to fully recover.

Two primary types of radiation therapy are external beam radiation therapy and internal beam radiation, also called brachytherapy. In colon cancer, external beam radiation is much more common than internal beam radiation.

1Reference: About.com

## 2What is Breast Cancer

Breast cancer is a malignant (cancerous) growth that begins in the tissues of the breast. Cancer is a disease in which abnormal cells grow in an uncontrolled way. Breast cancer is the most common cancer in women, but it can also appear in men. In the U.S., it affects one in eight women.

**The Most common types of breast cancer are:**

- Ductal carcinoma (85 - 90% of all cases)
- Lobular carcinoma (8% of all cases)

**Invasive (Infiltrating) Breast Cancer**
Invasive, or infiltrating, breast cancer has the potential to

spread out of the original tumor site and invade other parts of your breast and body. There are several types and subtypes of invasive breast cancer.

**Less Common Are:**

- Inflammatory breast cancer (occurs in the skin)
- Paget's disease of the nipple

## Symptoms of Breast Cancer:

- A lump or a thickening in the breast or in the armpit
- A change of size or shape of the mature breast
- Nipple fluid (not milk) leaking
- A change of size or shape of the nipple
- A change of color or texture of the nipple or the areloa, or of the skin of the breast itself (dimples,        puckers, rash)
- More details about symptoms of breast cancer.

**If You Have Breast Pain**
Early stages of breast cancer may not cause any pain or discomfort. Having a regular mammogram and a clinical breast exam by your health professional can help you understand changes in your breasts. Doing your breast self-exam can help you keep track of regular monthly changes.

Remember, many lumps and rashes are benign (not cancerous) and can respond well to proper treatment. If you experience any symptoms that cause you concern, see your doctor.

Treatments for breast cancer, as well as survival rates, are improving. Early detection and medical help is critical to improving the chances of living beyond a diagnosis of breast cancer.

# Breast Cancer in Men

3Even though men don't have breasts like women, they do have a small amount of breast tissue. The "breasts" of an adult man are similar to the breasts of a girl before puberty. In girls, this tissue grows and develops, but in men, it doesn't.  But because it is still breast tissue, men can get breast cancer. Men get the same types of breast cancers that women do, but cancers involving the parts that make and store milk are rare.

## Why Don't I Hear About Breast Cancer in Men as Much as I Hear About Breast Cancer in Women?

Even though men don't have breasts like women, they do have a small amount of breast tissue. The "breasts" of an adult man are similar to the breasts of a girl before puberty. In girls, this tissue grows and develops, but in men, it doesn't.

But because it is still breast tissue, men can get breast cancer. Men get the same types of breast cancers that women do, but cancers involving the parts that make and store milk are rare.

## Which Men Are More Likely to Get Breast Cancer?

It is rare for a man under age 35 to get breast cancer. The chance of a man getting breast cancer goes up with age. Most breast cancers happen to men between the ages of 60 and 70. Other risk factors of male breast cancer include:

- Breast cancer in a close female relative
- History of radiation exposure of the chest
- Enlargement of breasts (called gynecomastia) from drug or hormone treatments, or even
  some infections and poisons.
- Taking estrogen

- A rare genetic condition called Klinefelter's syndrome
- Severe liver disease (called cirrhosis)
- Diseases of the testicles such as mumps orchitis, a testicular injury, or an undescended
    testicle.

## How Serious Is Breast Cancer in Men?

Doctors used to think that breast cancer in men was more severe than it was in women, but it now seems that it's about the same.

The major problem is that breast cancer in men is often diagnosed later than breast cancer in women. This may be because men are less likely to be suspicious of something strange in that area. Also, their small amount of breast tissue is harder to feel, making it harder to catch these cancers early. It also means tumors can spread more quickly to surrounding tissues.

## What Are the Symptoms of Breast Cancer in Men?

Symptoms of breast cancer in men are similar to those in women. Most male breast cancers are diagnosed when a man discovers a lump on his chest. But unlike women, men tend to delay going to the doctor until they have more severe symptoms, like bleeding from the nipple. At that point the cancer may have already spread.

## How Is Breast Cancer Diagnosed and Treated in Men?

The same techniques that are used to diagnose breast cancer in women are used in men: physical exams, mammography, and biopsies (examining small samples of tissue under a microscope).

Likewise, the same treatments that are used in treating breast cancer in women -- surgery, radiation, chemotherapy, biological therapy, and hormone therapy -- are also used to treat breast cancer in men. The one major difference is that men with breast cancer respond much better to hormone therapy than women do. About 77% of male breast cancers have hormone receptors, meaning that hormone therapy can work in most men to treat the cancer.

3Reference:  WebMD Medical Reference
Reviewed by Angela Jain on April 14, 2014
© 2014 WebMD, LLC. All rights reserved.

# *Healing Scriptures*

# Healing Scriptures

Romans 10 tell us that faith comes from hearing and hearing from the word of Christ. To help us believe God for healing ourselves, our friends and our families it helps to have a good grasp of the Scriptures concerning healing. These Scriptures are small enough to be written on a business card or a small piece of paper, carried around and memorized.

**1.** (Exodus 15:26 NKJV) and said, If you diligently heed the voice of the LORD your God and do what is right in His sight, give ear to His commandments and keep all His statutes, I will put none of the diseases on you which I have brought on the Egyptians. For I am the LORD who heals you.

**2.** (Deuteronomy 32:39 NKJV) Now see that I, even I, am He, And there is no God besides Me; I kill and I make alive; I wound and I heal; Nor is there any who can deliver from My hand.

**3.** (2 Chronicles 7:14 NKJV) If My people who are called by My name will humble themselves, and pray and seek My face, and turn from their wicked ways, then I will hear from heaven, and will forgive their sin and heal their land.

**4.** (Psalms 30:2 NKJV) O LORD my God, I cried out to You, And You healed me.

**5.** (Psalms 6:2 NKJV) Have mercy on me, O LORD, for I am weak; O LORD, heal me, for my bones are troubled.

**6.** (Psalms 103:1-4 NKJV) Bless the LORD, O my soul; And all that is within me, bless His holy name! {2} Bless the LORD, O my soul, And forget not all His benefits: {3}

Who forgives all your iniquities, Who heals all your
diseases, {4} Who redeems your life from destruction,
Who crowns you with lovingkindness and tender mercies,

**7.** (Psalms 107:20 NKJV) He sent His word and healed
them, And delivered them from their destructions.

**8.** (Psalms 147:3 NKJV) He heals the brokenhearted And
binds up their wounds.

**9.** (Proverbs 3:7-8 NKJV) Do not be wise in your own
eyes; Fear the LORD and depart from evil. {8} It will be
health to your flesh, And strength to your bones.

**10.** (Proverbs 4:20-22 NKJV) My son, give attention to my
words; Incline your ear to my sayings. {21} Do not let
them depart from your eyes; Keep them in the midst of
your heart; {22} For they are life to those who find them,
And health to all their flesh.

**11.** (Isaiah 53:5 NKJV) But He was wounded for our
transgressions, He was bruised for our iniquities; The
chastisement for our peace was upon Him, And by His
stripes we are healed.

**12.** (Isaiah 58:8 NKJV) Then your light shall break forth
like the morning, Your healing shall spring forth speedily,
And your righteousness shall go before you; The glory of
the LORD shall be your rear guard.

**13.** (Isaiah 61:1 NKJV) "The Spirit of the Lord GOD is
upon Me, Because the LORD has anointed Me To preach
good tidings to the poor; He has sent Me to heal the
brokenhearted, To proclaim liberty to the captives, And the
opening of the prison to those who are bound;

**14.** (Jeremiah 3:22 NKJV) "Return, you backsliding children, And I will heal your backslidings." "Indeed we do come to You, For You are the LORD our God.

**15.** (Jeremiah 17:14 NKJV) Heal me, O LORD, and I shall be healed; Save me, and I shall be saved, For You are my praise.

**16.** (Jeremiah 30:17 NKJV) For I will restore health to you And heal you of your wounds,' says the LORD, 'Because they called you an outcast saying: "This is Zion; No one seeks her.
**17.** (Jeremiah 33:6 NKJV) 'Behold, I will bring it health and healing; I will heal them and reveal to them the abundance of peace and truth.

**18.** (Hosea 6:1 NKJV) Come, and let us return to the LORD; For He has torn, but He will heal us; He has stricken, but He will bind us up.

**19.** (Hosea 14:4 NKJV) I will heal their backsliding, I will love them freely, For My anger has turned away from him.

**20.** (Malachi 4:2 NKJV) But to you who fear My name The Sun of Righteousness shall arise With healing in His wings; And you shall go out And grow fat like stall-fed calves.

**21.** (Matthew 4:23 NKJV) And Jesus went about all Galilee, teaching in their synagogues, preaching the gospel of the kingdom, and healing all kinds of sickness and all kinds of disease among the people.

**22.** (Matthew 8:13 NKJV) Then Jesus said to the centurion, Go your way; and as you have believed, so let it be done for you. And his servant was healed that same hour.

**23.** (Matthew 8:16 NKJV) When evening had come, they brought to Him many who were demon-possessed. And He cast out the spirits with a word, and healed all who were sick.

**24.** (Matthew 9:35 NKJV) Then Jesus went about all the cities and villages, teaching in their synagogues, preaching the gospel of the kingdom, and healing every sickness and every disease among the people.

**25.** (Matthew 10:1 NKJV) And when He had called His twelve disciples to Him, He gave them power over unclean spirits, to cast them out, and to heal all kinds of sickness and all kinds of disease.

**26.** (Matthew 10:8 NKJV) Heal the sick, cleanse the lepers, raise the dead, cast out demons. Freely you have received, freely give.

**27.** (Matthew 12:22 NKJV) Then one was brought to Him who was demon-possessed, blind and mute; and He healed him, so that the blind and mute man both spoke and saw.

**28.** (Matthew 14:14 NKJV) And when Jesus went out He saw a great multitude; and He was moved with compassion for them, and healed their sick.

**29.** (Luke 6:19 NKJV) And the whole multitude sought to touch Him, for power went out from Him and healed them all.

**30.** (Luke 9:6 NKJV) So they departed and went through the towns, preaching the gospel and healing everywhere.(The twelve are sent out)

**31.** (Luke 10:8-9 NKJV) "Whatever city you enter, and

they receive you, eat such things as are set before you. {9} "And heal the sick there, and say to them, 'The kingdom of God has come near to you.'(The seventy are sent out)

**32.** (Luke 17:15 NKJV) And one of them, when he saw that he was healed, returned, and with a loud voice glorified God,(The story of the ten lepers)

**33.** (Acts 3:12 NKJV) So when Peter saw it, he responded to the people: "Men of Israel, why do you marvel at this? Or why look so intently at us, as though by our own power or godliness we had made this man walk?

**34.** (Healing of the lame man at the Gate Beautiful) (Acts 4:29-31 NKJV) "Now, Lord, look on their threats, and grant to Your servants that with all boldness they may speak Your word, {30} "by stretching out Your hand to heal, and that signs and wonders may be done through the name of Your holy Servant Jesus." {31} And when they had prayed, the place where they were assembled together was shaken; and they were all filled with the Holy Spirit, and they spoke the word of God with boldness.

**35.** (1 Corinthians 12:9 NKJV) to another faith by the same Spirit, to another gifts of healings by the same Spirit,

**36.** (James 5:14-16 NKJV) Is anyone among you sick? Let him call for the elders of the church, and let them pray over him, anointing him with oil in the name of the Lord. {15} And the prayer of faith will save the sick, and the Lord will raise him up. And if he has committed sins, he will be forgiven. {16} Confess your trespasses to one another, and pray for one another, that you may be healed. The effective, fervent prayer of a righteous man avails much.

**37.** (Revelation 22:2 NKJV) In the middle of its street, and

on either side of the river, was the tree of life, which bore
twelve fruits, each tree yielding its fruit every month. The
leaves of the tree were for the healing of the nations.

**38.** (Luke 8:47 NKJV) Now when the woman saw that she
was not hidden, she came trembling;
and falling down before Him, she declared to Him in the
presence of all the people the reason she had touched Him
and how she was healed immediately.

**39.** (Luke 8:48 NKJV) And He said to her, "Daughter, be
of good cheer; your faith has made you well. Go in peace."

**40.** (Luke 5:17 NKJV) Now it happened on a certain day,
as He was teaching, that there were Pharisees and teachers
of the law sitting by, who had come out of every town of
Galilee, Judea, and Jerusalem. And the power of the Lord
was present to heal them.

Reference: Newtestament.org

# Cancer Fighting Foods

# Cancer-Fighting Foods

Make fruits, vegetables, beans and whole grains the biggest part of every meal. Use this list next time you visit the grocery store.

## Grains
Wild or brown rice (regular or instant)
Whole grain pasta
Lentils

## Bread
Whole grain bread, tortillas or buns

## Cereal
Bran flakes
Oatmeal

## Snacks
Popcorn
Whole grain tortilla chips or crackers
Hummus
Almonds (plain, unsalted)

## Condiments

Olive oil
Canola oil
Low-fat or fat-free salad dressing

## Spices

Turmeric

## Beverages

Juice (100% juice, no added sugar)
Green or white tea (tea bags or loose)

## Produce

Sweet potatoes
Broccoli
Cauliflower
Brussels sprouts
Bok choy
Spinach (preferably organic)
Kale or collard greens (preferably organic)
Peas (fresh or frozen)
Romaine lettuce
Edamame
Tomatoes (no salt added if canned)
Garlic
Pears
Oranges
Red or purple grapes (preferably organic)
Fresh or frozen berries (preferably organic)

## Protein

Lean chicken or turkey
Lean fish such as salmon, halibut,
Redfish or Red snapper

Tofu
Black, red or pinto beans (low sodium)
Garbanzo beans/chickpeas (low sodium)

## Dairy
Skim milk
Low-fat cheese
Eggs or egg substitutes

## Vitamin D
This fat-soluble vitamin which helps absorb calcium to build strong teeth and bones may also build protection against cancer.

**High-fiber, cancer-fighting foods**

| | |
|---|---|
| **Whole grains** | whole-wheat pasta, raisin bran, barley, oatmeal, oat bran muffins, popcorn, brown rice, whole-grain or whole-wheat bread |
| **Fruit** | raspberries, apples, pears, strawberries, bananas, blackberries, blueberries, mango, apricots, citrus fruits, dried fruit, prunes, raisins |
| **Legumes** | lentils, black beans, split peas, lima beans, baked beans, kidney beans, pinto, chick peas, navy beans, black-eyed peas |
| **Vegetables** | broccoli, spinach, dark green leafy vegetables, peas, artichokes, corn, carrots, tomatoes, Brussels sprouts, potatoes |

Reference: www.mdanderson.org/prevention
Public Education Office

# Family Vacation

# Our Florida Vacation
# The Love of A Family is Life's
# Greatest Blessings

Despite what I was going through and how I was feeling I enjoyed my family and our family vacation. My family was my strength.

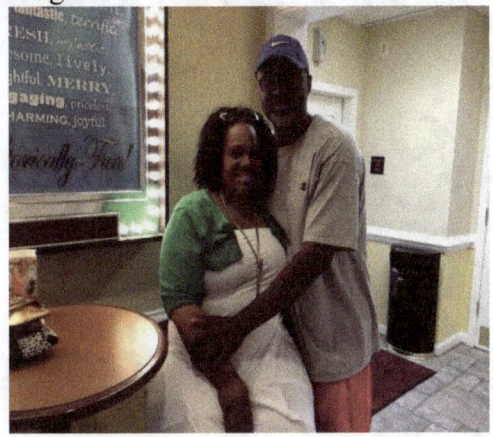

**Enjoying the resort where we stayed, watching the Disney fire works from the balcony**

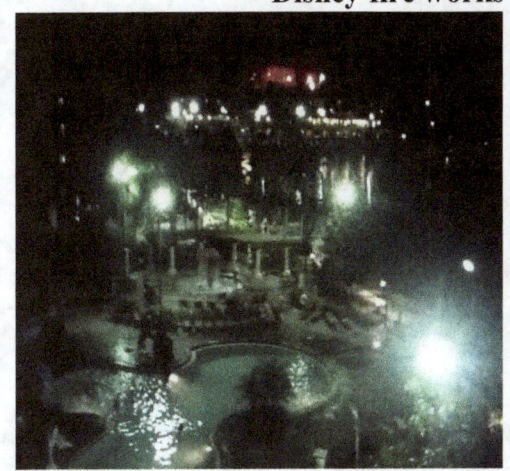
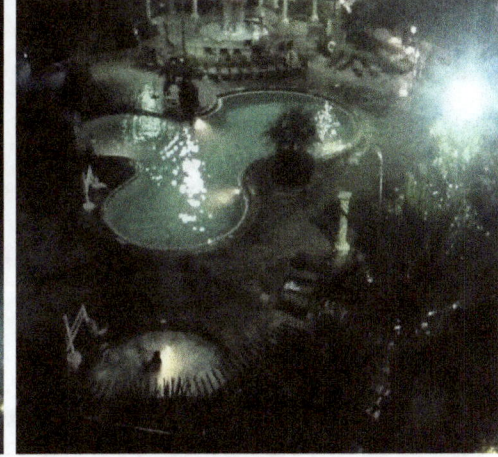

# The Many Faces of Chemo-Therapy

# The Many Faces of Chemotherapy

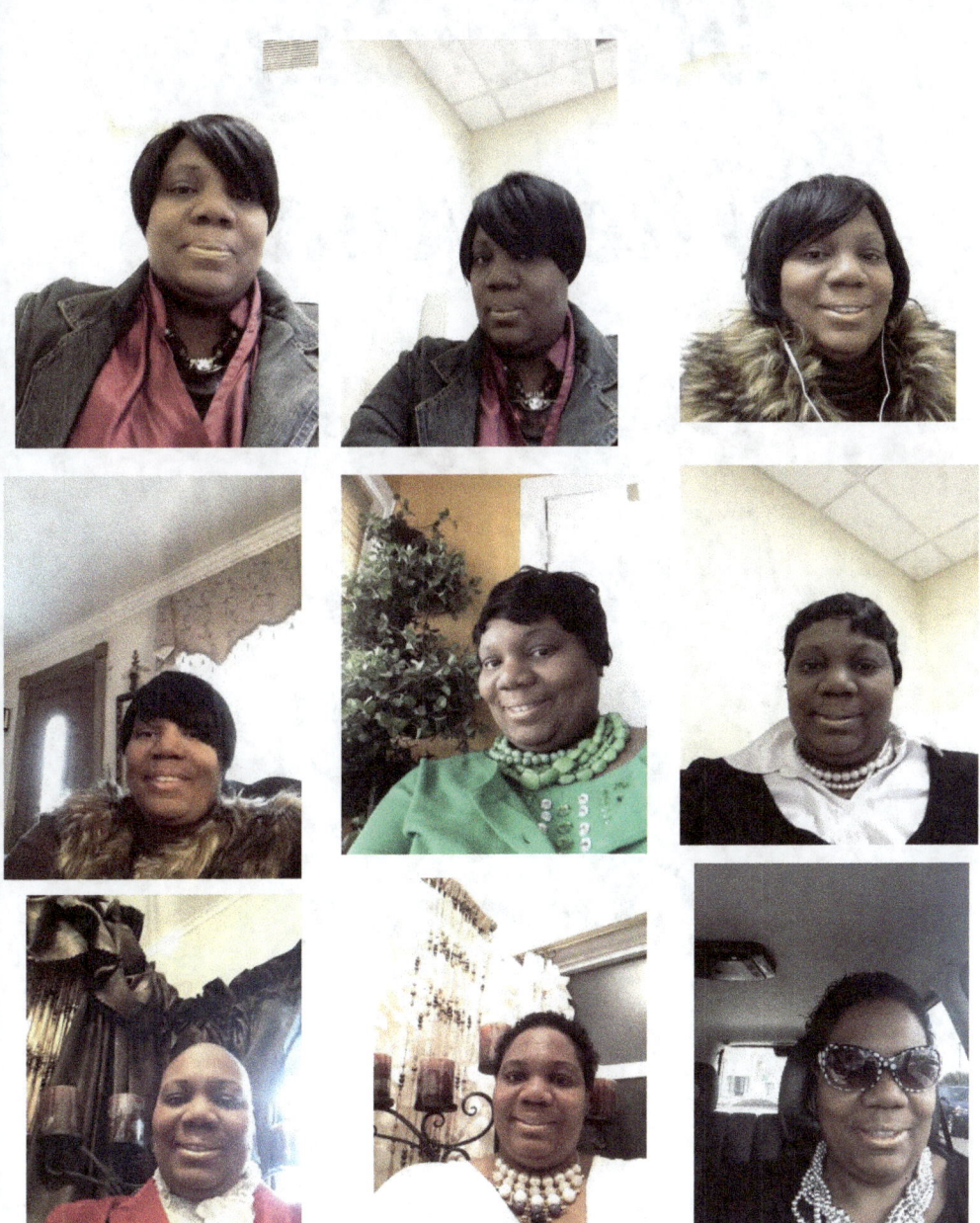

# Honoring The Man, The Legend, My Pastor Bishop W.L. Bonner

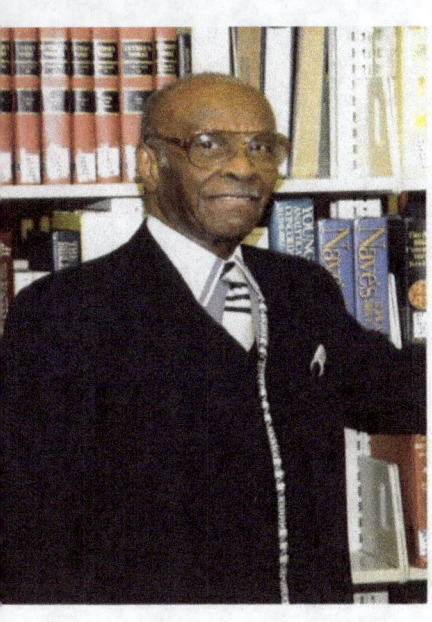

## My Pastor,
## The Late Bishop William
## Lee Bonner

I thank God every day for an amazing Pastor, the late Bishop William Lee Bonner. He was a true man of God who believed in the power of prayer. He often spoke from Deuteronomy 28:1-14, "The Blessing Plan". Those teachings resonated when I was going through my medical ordeal. Bishop William Bonner was a man of prayer; he would lay prostrate before God daily for the people of God. He not only prayed for you, he prayed for me. He taught me that prayer was essential and through prayer you gain access to God.

I thank God for his prayer life, his teachings, his faith and his integrity. What a blessing he has been to me and my family. I appreciate the Man, My Pastor, The Legend, Bishop William Lee Bonner.

I will see you in glory on that glorious day!!

# Prayer Warriors

James 5:14
Is any sick among you? let him call for the elders of the
church; and let them pray over him, anointing him with oil
in the name of the Lord..

## My Prayer Warriors During My Ordeal

I thank God every day for these amazing people. They have been such a blessing to me and my family. Their prayers have really bought me through.

My Assistant Pastor Bishop Charles E. & Faye Wright who have prayed with me and the family and who took time out of their busy schedule to come and administer communion to me.

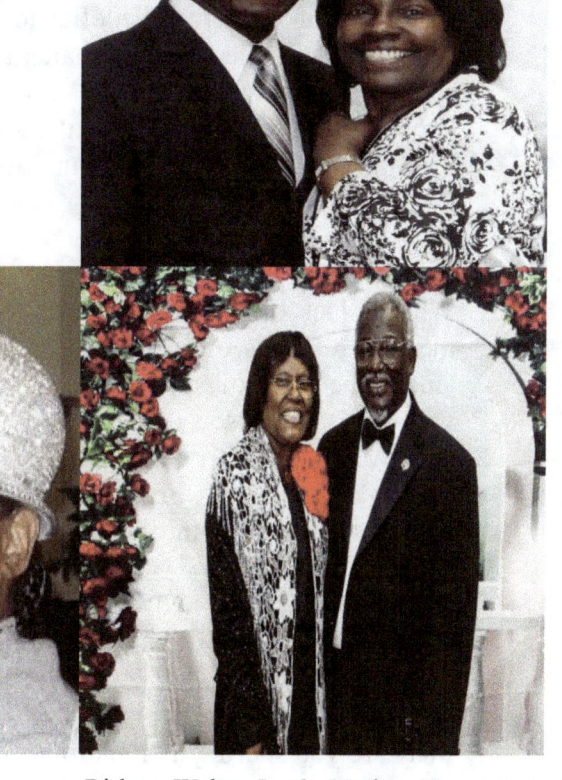

My other Pastor and Mother Bishop Wilbur & Mother Sandra Jones who called and continue to call to give encouraging words and prayer.

Bishop Walter L. & Mother Margaret Jackson what would I do without Family, a praying family. They called and offered a word of encouragement and prayed for me and the family daily.

# Admiration of God and His Handiwork 2014

Sometimes we take things for granted. As I looked out the window on my way to work one day after my many treatments, I began to see God's handy work in the snow. The air is purified with the snow. God knows exactly what we need when we need it. I actually did a little research on snow and found out that snow helps in the following areas:

**Agriculture**
There are at least two benefits to snow storms. A snow layer insulates the roots of plants and the small creatures spending the winter in the ground from cold winter temperatures. It also benefits the same as rain, as it melts the moisture sinks into the ground for better plant growth in the spring.

**Economy**
When a lack of snow contributes to agricultural shortages, the end result is often that the prices for food will rise. Under the laws of supply and demand, a reduced supply will cause increased demand which then drives the price up. When we start seeing higher prices for basic food staples due to a lack of snow fall months earlier, it affects us in ways we don't initially expect.

When you really think of the big picture, we really shouldn't complain when it is time to break out the shovels, now should we?

Why are you sharing this Sharon, well if God can look after the plants of the earth what will our heavenly father do for us. Just like God takes care of the earth by ensuring that we have rain, snow, heat and the necessary things to survive He is surely able to take good care of us even in our storms of life. Even in a bad storm God will bring forth a beautiful rainbow with such an array of colors. And even in your storm God can bring you out looking more radiant than ever.

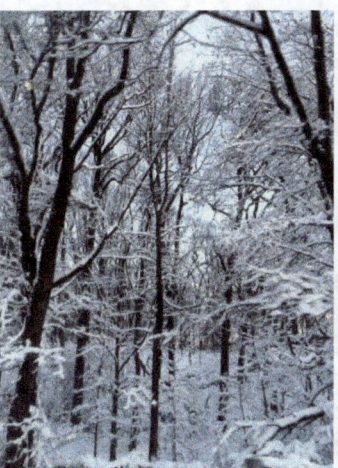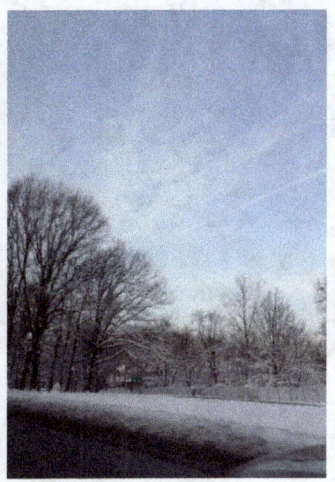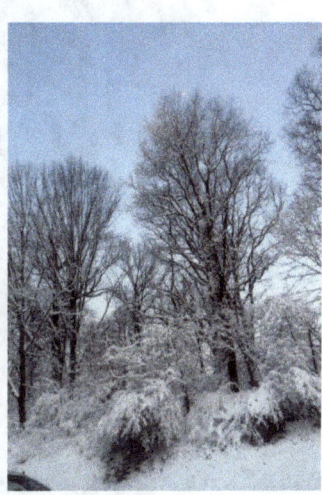

These are some beautiful pictures of God's handiwork. I want to encourage you that you are fearfully and wonderfully made. You are beautiful even when you are going through your struggle. **Psalm 139:14**
**I will praise thee; for I am fearfully and wonderfully made: marvelous are thy works; and that my soul knoweth right well.**

# The Strength of Family Runs Deep!

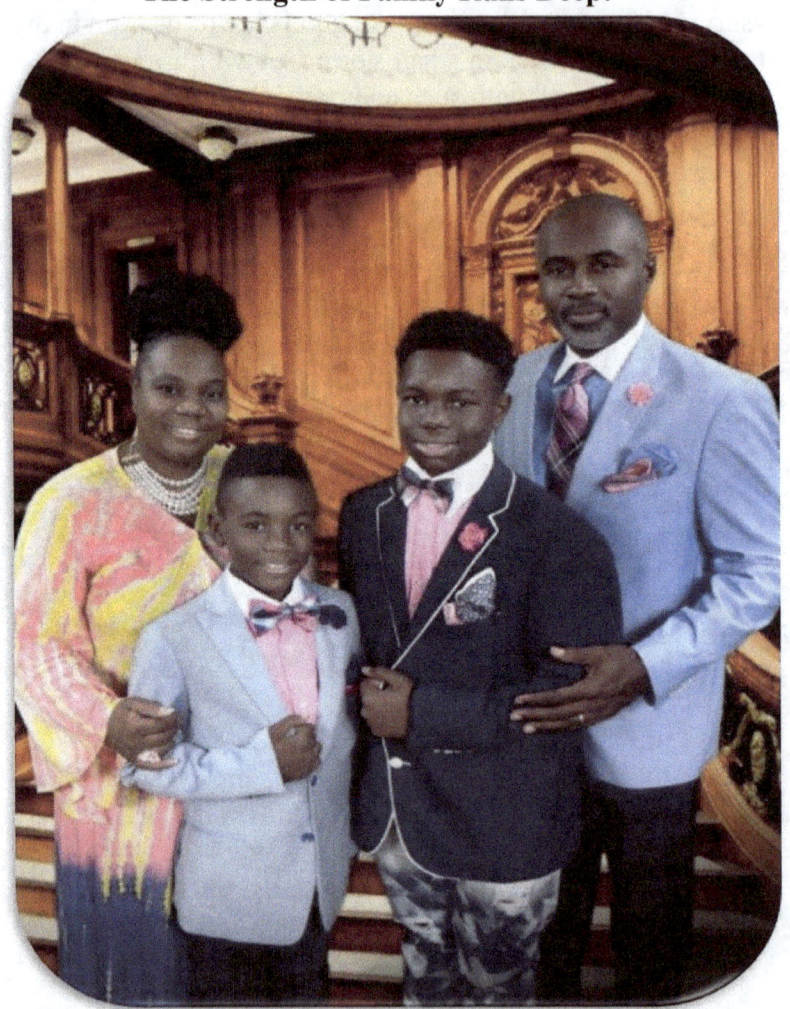

**Deuteronomy 28:4**
Blessed shall be the fruit of thy body, and the fruit of
thy ground, and the fruit of thy cattle, the increase of
thy kine, and the flocks of thy sheep.

**To God Be the Glory For The Things He Has Done!**

www.ingramcontent.com/pod-product-compliance
Lightning Source LLC
Chambersburg PA
CBHW060455290526
45791CB00001B/134